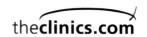

FOOT AND ANKLE CLINICS

Ankle Arthritis

GUEST EDITOR
Steven M. Raikin, MD

CONSULTING EDITOR
Mark S. Myerson, MD

September 2008 • Volume 13 • Number 3

SAUNDERS

An Imprint of Elsevier, Inc.
PHILADELPHIA   LONDON   TORONTO   MONTREAL   SYDNEY   TOKYO

W.B. SAUNDERS COMPANY
A Division of Elsevier Inc.

1600 John F. Kennedy Blvd., Suite 1800, Philadelphia, PA 19103-2899

http://www.theclinics.com

FOOT AND ANKLE CLINICS
September 2008
Editor: Debora Dellapena

Volume 13, Number 3
ISSN 1083-7515
ISBN-10: 1-4160-6295-5
ISBN-13: 978-1-4160-6295-0

Foot and Ankle Clinics (ISSN 1083-7515) is published quarterly by Elsevier, Inc., 360 Park Avenue South, New York, NY 10010-1710. Months of issue are March, June, September, and December. Business and Editorial Offices: 1600 John F. Kennedy Blvd., Suite 1800, Philadelphia, PA 19103-2899. Customer Service Office: 6277 Sea Harbor Drive, Orlando, FL 32887-4800. Periodicals postage paid at New York, NY, and additional mailing offices. Subscription prices are $345.00 per year Institutional, $297.00 per year Institutional USA, $345.00 per year Institutional Canada, $283.00 per year Personal, $209.00 per year Personal USA, $234.00 per year Personal Canada, $136.00 per year Personal student, $105.00 per year Personal student USA, $136.00 per year Personal student Canada. To receive student/resident rate, orders must be accompanied by name of affiliated institution, date of term, and the *signature* of program/residency coordinator on institution letterhead. Orders will be billed at individual rate until proof of status is received. Foreign air speed delivery is included in all *Clinics* subscription prices. All prices are subject to change without notice. POSTMASTER: Send address changes to *Foot and Ankle Clinics*, Elsevier Periodicals Customer Service, 6277 Sea Harbor Drive, Orlando, FL 32887-4800. **Customer Service: 1-800-654-2452 (US). From outside of the US, call 1- 407-563-6020. Fax: 1-407-363-9661. E-mail: JournalsCustomerService-usa@elsevier.com.**

Reprints. For copies of 100 or more of articles in this publication, please contact the Commercial Reprints Department, Elsevier Inc., 360 Park Avenue South, New York, NY 10010-1710. Tel.: 212-633-3812; Fax: 212-462-1935; E-mail: reprints@elsevier.com.

Printed in the United States of America.

CONSULTING EDITOR

MARK S. MYERSON, MD, Director, Institute for Foot and Ankle Reconstruction, Mercy Medical Center, Baltimore, Maryland

GUEST EDITOR

STEVEN M. RAIKIN, MD, Director, Orthopaedic Foot and Ankle Service, Rothman Institute; and Associate Professor, Orthopaedic Surgery, Jefferson Medical College, Philadelphia, Pennsylvania

CONTRIBUTORS

JAMAL AHMAD, MD, Assistant Professor, Rothman Institute Orthopaedics at Thomas Jefferson University Hospital, Philadelphia, Pennsylvania

JUDITH F. BAUMHAUER, MD, Professor, Department of Orthopaedics, Division of Foot and Ankle Surgery, University of Rochester Medical Center, Rochester, New York

TAMIR BLOOM, MD, Assistant Professor, Division of Pediatric Orthopaedics, Department of Orthopaedic Surgery, New Jersey Medical School University of Medicine and Dentistry of New Jersey, Newark, New Jersey

ERIC M. BLUMAN, MD, PhD, Director, Foot and Ankle Surgery, Division of Orthopaedic Surgery, Madigan Army Medical Center, Tacoma, Washington; Assistant Professor, Uniformed Services University of the Health Sciences, Bethesda, Maryland

REBECCA CERRATO, MD, The Institute for Foot and Ankle Reconstruction at Mercy, Mercy Medical Center, Baltimore, Maryland

WEN CHAO, MD, Department of Orthopaedic Surgery, University of Pennsylvania, Philadelphia, Pennsylvania

CHRISTOPHER P. CHIODO, MD, Director, Foot and Ankle Service, Department of Orthopaedic Surgery, Brigham and Women's Hospital, Boston, Massachusetts

J. CHRIS COETZEE, MD, Adjunct Associate Professor, Department of Orthopedics, University of Minnesota; and Minnesota Sports Medicine and Twin Cities Orthopedics, Minneapolis, Eden Prairie, Minnesota

TIM DANIELS, MD, FRCSC, Associate Professor, Foot and Ankle Surgery, Trauma, St. Michael's Hospital, University of Toronto, Toronto, Ontario, Canada

MICHAEL S. HENNESSY, BSc, FRCSEd (Tr&Orth), Consultant Orthopaedic Surgeon, Department of Orthopaedics, Wirral University Hospitals NHS Trust, Upton, Wirral, United Kingdom

CLIFFORD L. JENG, MD, Institute for Foot and Ankle Reconstruction, Mercy Medical Center, Baltimore, Maryland

SHAUN K. KHOSLA, MD, Resident Physician, Department of Orthopaedics, University of Rochester Medical Center, Rochester, New York

BRADLEY M. LAMM, DPM, Head of the Podiatry Section, International Center for Limb Lengthening, Rubin Institute for Advanced Orthopedics, Sinai Hospital of Baltimore, Baltimore, Maryland

SHELDON S. LIN, MD, Associate Professor, Foot and Ankle Division, Department of Orthopaedic Surgery, New Jersey Medical School University of Medicine and Dentistry of New Jersey, Newark, New Jersey

ANDREW P. MOLLOY, FRCS (Tr&Orth), Consultant Orthopaedic Surgeon, Department of Orthopaedics, University Hospital Aintree, Liverpool, United Kingdom

MARK S. MYERSON, MD, Director, Institute for Foot and Ankle Reconstruction, Mercy Medical Center, Baltimore, Maryland

DROR PALEY, MD, FRCSC, Director, International Center for Limb Lengthening, Rubin Institute for Advanced Orthopedics, Sinai Hospital of Baltimore; Consultant for Smith & Nephew, Baltimore, Maryland

MURRAY PENNER, MD, FRCSC, Clinical Assistant Professor, Department of Orthopaedics, University of British Columbia, Vancouver, Canada

RACHANA M. PUROHIT, DPM, Clinical Fellow, International Center for Limb Lengthening, Rubin Institute for Advanced Orthopedics, Sinai Hospital of Baltimore, Baltimore, Maryland

STEVEN M. RAIKIN, MD, Director, Orthopaedic Foot and Ankle Service, Rothman Institute; and Associate Professor, Orthopaedic Surgery, Jefferson Medical College, Philadelphia, Pennsylvania

VENKAT RAMPURI, MD, Orthopaedic Resident, Department of Orthopaedic Surgery, Jefferson Medical College, Thomas Jefferson University Hospital, Philadelphia, Pennsylvania

REGIS RENARD, MD, Resident, Department of Orthopaedic Surgery, New Jersey Medical School University of Medicine and Dentistry of New Jersey, Newark, New Jersey

STACY C. SPECHT, MPA, Research Manager, International Center for Limb Lengthening, Rubin Institute for Advanced Orthopedics, Sinai Hospital of Baltimore, Baltimore, Maryland

RHYS THOMAS, FRCS(Orth) FFSEM(UK), Consultant Orthopaedic Surgeon, University Hospital of Wales, Cardiff, United Kingdom

KEITH WAPNER, MD, Department of Orthopaedic Surgery, University of Pennsylvania, Philadelphia, Pennsylvania

KEVIN WING, MD, FRCSC, Clinical Assistant Professor, Department of Orthopaedics, University of British Columbia, Vancouver, Canada

HUGH Y. WON, MBBS, Institute for Foot and Ankle Reconstruction, Mercy Medical Center, Baltimore, Maryland

EDWARD V. WOOD, FRCS (Tr&Orth), Foot and Ankle Fellow, Department of Orthopaedics, Wirral University Hospitals NHS Trust, Upton, Wirral, United Kingdom

PRAVEEN YALAMANCHILI, MD, Resident, Department of Orthopaedic Surgery, New Jersey Medical School University of Medicine and Dentistry of New Jersey, Newark, New Jersey

ALASTAIR S.E. YOUNGER, MD, MB, ChB, FRCSC, Clinical Associate Professor, Department of Orthopaedics, University of British Columbia, Vancouver, Canada

CONTENTS

Of all joints in the body, the ankle joint is subjected to the highest forces per square centimeter and is injured more commonly. Yet, the incidence of symptomatic ankle arthritis is much lower than that of the knee and hip. Various mechanical, biochemical and anatomic peculiarities of the ankle account for its apparent resilience to the process of aging and trauma. The goal of this article is to help the reader better understand the functional paradoxes that make the ankle joint a unique and fascinating articulation.

Glucosamine and chondroitin sulfate are the most well-marketed dietary supplements directed toward managing symptoms associated with osteoarthritis. The presumption of their benefit in the ankle is based largely on promising results from their use in knee osteoarthritis. Likewise, viscosupplementation has proved to be efficacious in the management of osteoarthritis of the knee. Preliminary studies demonstrate a realization of this benefit in the ankle joint, but further research is required. So far, the literature has shown the dietary and viscosupplementation discussed in this article to be relatively safe for use.

on the various design characteristics of the different mobile-bearing designs and reviews the outcome research to date.

Management of Varus or Valgus Ankle Deformity with Ankle Replacement

J. Chris Coetzee

Ankle replacements are probably here to stay. Improved designs and surgical technique led to much better mid-term and longer term outcomes than the first-generation replacements in the 1970s. Multiple recent papers also have discussed the many potential complications with total ankle replacement surgery. As we proceed in the future, one should be cognizant of all the pitfalls and know how to deal with the difficult ankles, especially varus and valgus deformities. There should be a clear understanding that the greater the varus or valgus, the harder the procedure and the less predictable the outcome of ankle replacement.

Primary and Revision Total Ankle Replacement Using Custom-Designed Prostheses

Mark S. Myerson and Hugh Y. Won

With means for better mechanical stability and fixation, custom prostheses have improved our capabilities in salvaging failed total ankle replacements. Even in the primary total ankle replacement setting, previous contraindications due to suboptimal bony support may be adequately bypassed, and more patients may benefit from having a custom prosthesis. Accurate preoperative imaging and templating will ensure proper dimensions of the custom prosthesis. Intraoperative adjuncts such as screws, plates, and bone grafts will help address unexpected bone defects, coexisting adjacent joints arthritis, and other hindfoot and midfoot deformities. In this article, the authors discuss the history and problems of total ankle replacement failures, the surgical technique, and tips and pitfalls when using custom replacement prostheses.

Allograft Total Ankle Replacement—A Dead Ringer to the Natural Joint

Clifford L. Jeng and Mark S. Myerson

For decades, orthopedic surgeons have been looking for practical alternatives to ankle arthrodesis for the treatment of end-stage ankle arthritis. The most popular alternatives available today are total ankle replacement, supramalleolar osteotomy, and ankle distraction arthroplasty. Fresh bipolar osteochondral allograft of the ankle joint has been sporadically reported in the literature as another alternative to ankle fusion. This article examines the basic science supporting the use of this technique, discusses the five case series reported in the literature, and describes the authors' preferred technique and short-term results.

Index

FORTHCOMING ISSUES

RECENT ISSUES

ELSEVIER
SAUNDERS

Foot Ankle Clin N Am
13 (2008) xiii–xiv

FOOT AND
ANKLE CLINICS

Foreword

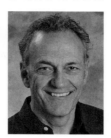

Mark S. Myerson, MD
Consulting Editor

Where are we headed with the treatment of ankle arthritis? There has been such an evolution in the understanding of the biology and treatment of arthritis by both medical and mechanical means during the past few decades. I wonder what our treatment alternatives will be in the future? Have you encountered the patient who asks "What is the current newest technology for treatment of ankle arthritis" or "What is on the horizon over the next few years in treatment?" For many patients, treatment of end-stage arthritis remains either an arthrodesis or a joint replacement. Other patients may be candidates for an interim type of treatment, for example with a tibial osteotomy or a distraction arthroplasty. I use the term "interim treatment" because the benefit may not be long lasting, but the treatment may play an essential role in improving symptoms and delaying the need for either arthrodesis or arthroplasty.

Logically, a biologic type of treatment for ankle arthritis would be ideal, and this goal prompted many surgeons to perform an osteoarticular allograft replacement. Unfortunately, although the early reported results were promising, the failure rate is high, and one must consider carefully which patients are suitable for this type of treatment, because salvage of a failed allograft replacement can be difficult. Of note, there is no discussion of arthroscopy in the management of ankle arthritis in this issue. Although there may be a role for arthroscopy as an adjunct to treatment with osteotomy or distraction, the long-term results do not warrant arthroscopy as the sole treatment for ankle arthritis.

doi:10.1016/j.fcl.2008.06.001

This is an exciting issue of *Foot and Ankle Clinics* and should be a tremendous help to the surgeon interested in the management of primary and tertiary deformity of the ankle.

Mark S. Myerson, MD
Institute for Foot and Ankle Reconstruction
Mercy Medical Center
301 St Paul Place
Baltimore, MD, 21202

E-mail address: Mark4feet@aol.com

Preface

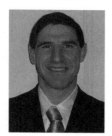

Steven M. Raikin, MD
Guest Editor

The tibiotalar (ankle) joint is one of the hardiest and arthritis-resistant joints in the body, rarely afflicted with primary osteoarthritis. When degenerative change occurs at the ankle joint it is most commonly because of trauma or abnormal ankle mechanics, or less commonly, inflammatory or neuropathic arthropathies. When arthritis does occur, the resultant physical disability and the effect on quality of life and mental well being are significant.

It has been a privilege to serve as the Guest Editor of this edition of *Foot and Ankle Clinics,* reviewing the current understanding of the biomechanics and management of ankle arthritis. Over the past decade, our understanding of this important topic has greatly evolved. New nonsurgical modalities are now available, which attempt to delay or reverse the cartilage degeneration orthobiologically, while joint-sparing surgical alternatives to fusions continue to stimulate discussion and research. Arthrodesis remains the current gold standard for the management of end-stage arthritis, with new concepts including minimally invasive approaches, salvage reconstruction, and conversion to joint arthroplasty. Since the Agility total ankle became the first new generation total ankle arthroplasty to gain Food and Drug Administration approval in 1999, more than a dozen arthroplasty systems have become available worldwide, and this number and our experience with them continues to grow.

For this issue I have invited an outstanding group of academically dedicated physicians from the United States, Canada, and the United Kingdom

1083-7515/08/$ - see front matter © 2008 Elsevier Inc. All rights reserved.
doi:10.1016/j.fcl.2008.05.004

to share their expertise on these topics. Through their incredible efforts I feel we have created an edition of *Foot and Ankle Clinics* that covers the spectrum of our most up-to-date knowledge about ankle arthritis and its management. I personally thank each of them for helping to create an outstanding addition to the literature regarding ankle arthritis.

Steven M. Raikin, MD
Director Orthopaedic Foot and Ankle Service
Rothman Institute and Jefferson University Hospital
925 Chestnut Street
Philadelphia, PA 19107, USA

Associate Professor Orthopaedic Surgery
Jefferson Medical College
111 S 11th Street
Philadelphia, PA 19107, USA

E-mail address: steven.raikin@rothmaninstitute.com

ELSEVIER
SAUNDERS

Foot Ankle Clin N Am
13 (2008) xvii

FOOT AND
ANKLE CLINICS

Dedication

I would like to dedicate this issue to my wife and children, and to the wives and children of each of the contributing authors, who sacrificed many hours and nights, allowing the time commitment required to write the articles for this edition.

Additionally, I dedicate this issue to Mark S. Myerson, a friend and mentor, and wish him health and the strength to continue for many years to come.

Steven M. Raikin, MD

1083-7515/08/$ - see front matter © 2008 Elsevier Inc. All rights reserved.
doi:10.1016/j.fcl.2008.05.003

foot.theclinics.com

ELSEVIER
SAUNDERS

Foot Ankle Clin N Am
13 (2008) 341–352

FOOT AND
ANKLE CLINICS

Etiology and Biomechanics of Ankle Arthritis

Tim Daniels, MD, FRCSC[a],*,
Rhys Thomas, FRCS(Orth) FFSEM(UK)[b]

[a]*Foot and Ankle Surgery, Trauma, St. Michael's Hospital, University of Toronto, Ste. 800,*
55 Queen Street East, Toronto, ON, Canada M5C 1R6
[b]*University Hospital of Wales, Cardiff, CF14 4XW, United Kingdom*

In an open kinetic chain, the foot minus the talus functions as a single fibro-osseous unit [1]. As a consequence, the ankle joint is the first major articulation responsible for transferring the ground reactive forces to the remainder of the body. The ankle joint is subjected to the highest forces per square centimeter and is injured more commonly than any other joint in the body. Yet, the incidence of symptomatic ankle arthritis is approximately nine times lower than that of the knee and hip [2–4]. Various mechanical, biochemical and anatomic peculiarities of the ankle account for its apparent resilience to the process of aging and trauma. The goal of this article is to help the reader better understand these functional paradoxes that make the ankle joint a unique and fascinating articulation.

Etiology and epidemiology of ankle arthritis

The ankle is one of the most arthritis-resistant joints in the body [5]. Unlike the hip and knee, the ankle joint rarely is affected by primary osteoarthritis. When degenerative change is present at the ankle joint, it is caused most commonly by trauma and/or abnormal ankle mechanics [6]. Less common causes include inflammatory arthropathies, hemochromatosis, or neuropathic arthropathy [7,8]. Ankle trauma precipitating arthritis can consist of fractures to the malleoli, tibial plafond, talus, or isolated osteochondral damage of the talar dome. Instability of the ankle caused by chronic lateral ligament laxity may lead to the development of osteoarthritis in the medial joint compartment [9].

---

* Corresponding author.
E-mail address: danielst@smh.toronto.on.ca (T. Daniels).

1083-7515/08/$ - see front matter © 2008 Elsevier Inc. All rights reserved.
doi:10.1016/j.fcl.2008.05.002

The reported incidence of post-traumatic arthritis after ankle fracture is variable. Although it is often difficult to predict the likelihood of developing post-traumatic osteoarthritis following an injury, several factors have been identified. The severity of the initial injury, indicated by the amount of disruption to the articular cartilage, is an important positive predictor for the development of ankle arthritis. Lindsjo reported a series of over 300 ankle fractures treated with open reduction and internal fixation [10]. In this series, the incidence of post-traumatic arthritis occurred in 14% of patients and was correlated directly to the fracture pattern. Using the Weber classification [11], the incidence of post-traumatic arthritis in type A ankle fractures was 4%; in type B, it was 12%, and in Type C it was 33%. Lindsjo's study supported the observations of others, whereby the presence a posterior malleolar fragment, even if small, indicated a more severe injury and an increased incidence of post-traumatic arthritis [12,13]. If the posterior fragment was surface-bearing (greater than 20% of the tibial plafond), the incidence of post-traumatic arthritis was 34%; with a small posterior fragment, the incidence was 17%, and with no posterior fragment, the incidence was 4%.

The results of Lindsjo's study [10] also indicated that the adequacy of reduction following a fracture is a strong determinant of outcome. A significantly greater proportion of patients who had nonanatomic reduction demonstrated radiographic changes of osteoarthritis then those who had rigid anatomic fixation. A strong correlation was seen between the degree of osteoarthritis on radiograph and clinical result. The benefit of anatomic reduction is not questioned, but debate remains as to whether similar results may be obtained from adequate closed versus open reduction. Lindsjo's series also demonstrated the worst overall results in women aged between 45 and 64 years. Following ankle fracture, radiological arthritic changes, if present, tend to occur within 2 years. Such changes may not progress, and symptoms may improve with time [10].

In fractures of the tibial plafond, a combination of initial trauma and avascular necrosis contributes to the development of post-traumatic arthritis. A direct correlation between adequacy of reduction and functional and radiographic outcome has been reported at long-term follow-up [14]. Regardless of reduction, the presence of chondral damage to the plafond or talus and avascular necrosis of subchondral bone increases the chances of subsequent arthritis [15,16]. This explains why AO type C1 and C2 fractures have much better outcomes than the more complex type C3 fractures regardless of treatment. Best outcome is forecast by minimal articular damage, anatomic reduction, early mobilization, and lack of complications. In his series of patients, Ruedi [14] noted that lack of joint arthrosis at 1 to 2 years forecasts a further absence for another 5 to 10 years.

Fractures of the talus, although rarer than ankle fractures, also may give rise to ankle arthritis. Following talar neck fractures, post-traumatic arthritis may be seen at both tibio–talar and subtalar joints, and it is caused by direct articular damage, subchondral collapse from avascular necrosis, or malunion causing abnormal joint mechanics. The incidence of arthritis varies from 47% to 97% [17].

Osteoarthritis can occur in 20% to 50% of patients who have osteochondral fractures of the talus. Joint degeneration is related to the size and location of the lesion, the patient's weight, and associated ligamentous laxity [18].

The pathogenesis of arthritis at the ankle appears to be different to that at the hip or knee. The reason for this discrepancy becomes evident when the mechanics and biology of the ankle joint are considered.

The ankle moves mainly as a rolling joint and exhibits congruency at high load, whereas the knee exhibits a combination of rolling, sliding, and rotation that may predispose it to a higher incidence of osteoarthritis [19]. Evidence supports the fact that ankle articular cartilage has distinct characteristics. Although these differences may help protect the ankle from primary osteoarthritis, they may increase its susceptibility to post-traumatic degeneration. In general, degenerative changes are related to biomechanical, molecular, or pathologic factors. Understanding the complex pathogenesis of joint osteoarthritis is important in allowing early detection of disease, determining treatment options, and possibly allowing disease modification.

Articular cartilage thickness

The thickness of articular cartilage affects the stresses and strains that arise in the cartilage matrix. Significant differences in articular cartilage thickness and uniformity are seen between the hip, knee, and ankle [20,21]. Shepherd and Seedhom [20] studied cartilage thickness in the joints of the lower limb. They found that in all specimens, the ankle had the thinnest cartilage, whereas the thickest was always in the knee. An inverse relationship also was found between cartilage thickness and its compressive modulus (ie, a thin ankle cartilage has a high compressive modulus). Ankle articular cartilage is relatively uniform in thickness, ranging from approximately 1 to 1.7 mm, whereas knee cartilage has been shown to have a large variation in thickness from 1 to 6 mm. Simon and colleagues [22] proposed that thickness of cartilage is related to joint congruency, with the most congruent joints having the thinnest cartilage that acts to equalize the stresses.

This view was shared by Wynarsky and Greenwald [23] from their work on a mathematical model of the ankle joint. They demonstrated a change in congruency in the ankle with change in load. They found that as pressure was increased, the load-bearing area changed from two localized areas to a much larger region. Under maximum physiologic loads, the joint transforms from incongruence to congruence and allows the resulting applied forces to be distributed over a large area; this, in turn, allows the joint to withstand large pressures efficiently. The change in congruity may have a beneficial effect on articular cartilage lubrication and nutrition, as well as dissipating force, thereby contributing to resistance from primary degeneration.

Articular contact area

Compared with the hip and knee, the articular surface area of the ankle joint is equivalent. The average cartilage coverage area of the tibia is 965 mm^2 and of the talus 1305 mm^2 [24]. In the loaded ankle joint, however, the area of articular surface contact between bearing surfaces is much smaller. At 500N load, the ankle has a contact area of 350 mm^2, as compared with 1100 mm^2 for the hip and 1120 mm^2 for the knee [25–27]. The average talocrural cartilage contact areas are minimal at heel strike (272 mm^2) and maximal at midstance (417 mm^2) [24]. Changes in contact stress and contact area may increase the probability of fatigue failure of the articular cartilage and may allow precipitation of post-traumatic arthritic change.

An in vitro investigation of such changes occurring after an injury has produced some confusion. The classic biomechanical study by Ramsey and Hamilton [28] demonstrated that a 1 mm lateral talar shift dramatically reduced the tibio–talar contact area and often was quoted to advocate anatomic stabilization of all ankle fractures. The methods used do not represent a physiologic state, because a constrained/static model was used, with the fibula being resected and the talus being forced into a displaced lateral position. Subsequent studies that have reproduced a static translation of the talus within the ankle mortise have supported Ramsey and Hamilton's original results [29,30].

Further studies using dynamic/unconstrained models have not reproduced the findings of Ramsey and Hamilton and have served to underline the fact that the medial structures are the primary stabilizers of the ankle joint. Clarke and colleagues [31] found that up to 6 mm of lateral displacement caused no significant difference in the tibio–talar contact area; however, when medial instability was produced by sectioning the deltoid ligament, the total contact area was decreased by 15% to 20%. Pereira and colleagues [32] demonstrated no significant effect of mortise widening on ankle contact area or talar shift. Curtis and colleagues [33] identified a 30% decrease in tibio–talar contact with 30° of external rotation and 2 mm of shortening of the fibula. The decrease in contact area doubled with sectioning of the deltoid ligament. These physiologic studies demonstrate that the primary stabilizers at the ankle joint are medial, and with a displaced fibular fracture, the talus tends not to follow the lateral fibular displacement maximally unless there is insufficiency of the deltoid ligament.

The difference in findings between these studies results from the fact that the ankle tends to assume a position of inherent stability when loaded. The ankle carries loads of up to five times the body weight on normal level walking [5] and loading leads to increased joint congruency.

Mechanical properties

Several studies have compared the biomechanical properties of human ankle cartilage with those of the hip and knee. Kempson [34] investigated the effect of aging on the mechanical properties of cartilage in the hip and ankle joints. The tensile properties of normal, intact cartilage were tested, and it was observed that the tensile fracture stress of the femoral head deteriorated considerably with age, while that of the talus did not. Based on previous work, it was postulated that this deterioration in tensile properties is related to disruption of the collagen fibril network by progressive fatigue. In contrast to the hip, tensile strength of the talus decreased only slightly with age and cartilage. Even in the eighth and ninth decades, it was strong enough to resist everyday physiologic stresses. This may be the mechanism by which the ankle joint resists primary osteoarthritic change.

Swann and Seedhom [35] measured indentation stiffness of normal articular cartilage of the knee and ankle and found ankle cartilage to be stiffer. A relationship between stiffness and estimated stresses experienced by the cartilage was suggested. It was postulated that areas subjected to high stress adapt by increasing in stiffness, whereas those areas that experience high stresses infrequently are most susceptible to developing arthritic changes. Topographic studies show cartilage material properties to be more uniform in the ankle than in the hip and knee [36].

Cyclical loading has been shown to alter chondrocyte metabolism [37]. As talar cartilage is more resistant to physiologic stresses, chondrocytes are affected less by normal aging. As such, chondrocytes would continue to synthesize the main constituents of cartilage. The higher stresses may occur in the ankle following trauma, which may lead to a change in chondrocyte metabolism, deterioration in collagen, and the subsequent development of osteoarthritis.

Recent work has drawn attention to the importance of the superficial layer of articular cartilage in the development of arthritic change [19,38]. Significant biomechanical and biochemical differences have been demonstrated between the superficial layers of normal knee and ankle cartilage. Compressive deformity of cartilage during cyclical loading is confined to the more superficial regions. As talar cartilage is thinner than cartilage from the knee, the superficial layer makes up a greater proportion of its thickness, and it is postulated that this may have a role in resisting osteoarthritic change [19]. It also appears that subchondral bone in the ankle is less responsive to alterations in load, as the increase in bone density seen in the subchondral layer of the severely arthritic knee is not seen in the degenerative ankle [38].

Articular cartilage metabolism

Although anatomic and biomechanical differences exist between the joints of the lower limb, these differences alone may not explain entirely the differences in susceptibility to arthritic change. The destructive process accompanying the development of osteoarthritis is mediated by matrix metalloproteinases (MMP). This family of substances is proteolytic to all known cartilage matrix components, including proteoglycans, collagens, noncollagenous proteins, and matrix glycoproteins. In studies on human tissues, it has been observed that MMP-8 is expressed by chondrocytes and is elevated in osteoarthritis cartilages [39,40].

Chubinskaya and colleagues [41] demonstrated that expression of MMP-8 was seen in knee cartilage but not in ankle cartilage unless the ankle cartilage showed degenerative change. MMP-8 expression was seen following the action of the catabolic cytokine, interleukin (IL)-1 beta on normal ankle cartilage. Recent study has suggested that some MMPs may play a role in normal cartilage homeostasis, with only the expression of some members (MMP-3, 8) being related to articular cartilage damage [42].

Kang and colleagues [43] demonstrated a significant difference in chondrocyte response to stimulation by fibronectin fragments. Knee chondrocytes showed greater proteoglycan (PG) loss and increased aggrecanase activity when compared with the ankle. Ankle cartilage was much more refractory to damage than knee cartilage from the same donor.

IL-1 beta is effective in inhibiting PG synthesis from chondrocytes of the knee and ankle [44]. The inhibitory response was much greater in the knee than in ankle chondrocytes and appears to be related to the numbers or types of receptors present on the chondrocytes. The effect of IL-1 was overcome more effectively by IL-1 receptor antagonist protein in the ankle than in the knee.

The pathogenesis of ankle osteoarthritis is a complex event to which anatomic, biomechanical, and metabolic factors may all contribute. All the joints of the lower limbs are subjected to similar loads during weight bearing [45], yet the incidence of osteoarthritis among these joints is quite variable. Such differences in the incidence of osteoarthritis and etiology of arthritis suggest that the ankle is more resistant to primary osteoarthritis but more susceptible to post-traumatic degeneration. The ankle may be protected from the development of primary osteoarthritis by its metabolic properties, tensile characteristics, uniformity, congruency, and restrained movement. The thinness of ankle articular cartilage and the high peak contact stresses to which it is submitted may make it less adaptable to the incongruity, decreased stability, or increased stresses that may follow a traumatic event.

Incidence of ankle arthritis

The true incidence of osteoarthritis in the ankle joint is difficult to determine mainly because of the variation between degenerative change and clinical correlation. Cadaveric, radiographic, and clinical studies all indicate that arthritis at the ankle is less common than at the knee or hip [2,4,46–48]. Epidemiologic studies show that 6% of the population is affected by knee osteoarthritis; this number increases to 10% in people aged over 65 years. Although symptomatic osteoarthritis does present at the ankle, it is rare even in the elderly. In clinical practice [2,4,46], patients who have symptomatic arthritis of the knee are seen about eight to nine times more commonly than those who have symptomatic arthritis of the ankle. It is estimated that knee replacement is performed about 25 times more frequently than either arthrodesis or arthroplasty of the ankle.

In the knee, fibrillation and full-thickness articular cartilage changes are believed to progress to osteoarthritis. Similar changes may be seen at the-ankle but may not progress in the same manner. Random autopsy studies of ankles and knees found full-thickness cartilage defects in 44% of knees and only 2% of ankles [48,49]. A further study [50] using a wider definition of the term degeneration reported 98% of ankles as having degenerative changes; Muehleman and colleagues [51] found 66% of knee joints to be osteoarthritic as compared with 18% of cadaveric ankles.

The frequency of degenerative changes reported in the ankle would be much higher than clinically expected if they all progressed to osteoarthritis. Koepp and colleagues [47] evaluated the prevalence of articular cartilage degeneration in cadaveric knee and ankle cartilage from donors who had no history of joint disease. Although the frequency of degenerative changes increased with age, a large number of knee and ankle joints were found to have no detectable degeneration, even in donors over the age of 60 years (38% of the ankle, 4% of the knee). In ankles where degenerative change was seen, disease of equal or greater severity was observed in the knee. This may suggest that joint degeneration is not as common a part of normal aging as previously thought and that changes described as preosteoarthritic may not progress in the same manner in the knee and ankle joints.

Ankle arthritis and gait mechanics

The foot and its articulations allow for a smooth transition of forces from the hindfoot to the forefoot with minimal energy expenditure. The ankle joint and the motion it provides in the sagittal plane play a pivotal role in the mechanics of gait. During steady- state walking, the foot functions as a three-rocker mechanism:

1. The heel functions as the first rocker during initial heel strike and the first 30% of the stance phase. During the initial portion of the stance phase, the ankle is plantarflexing such that the foot can contact the ground.
2. The ankle joint functions as the second rocker during the midportion of the stance phase and allows the body weight to be transferred effectively to the forefoot. This is the point in the gait cycle where maximum ankle dorsiflexion is attained. This smooth transfer of forces from the hindfoot to the forefoot only can occur if the midfoot is rigid.
3. The forefoot break functions as the third rocker during the latter portion of the stance phase with external rotation of the foot and leg during this phase in gait [53].

The primary motion of the ankle joint occurs in the sagittal plane. The average arc of ankle flexion and extension is 43° to 63°, and only 30° of this motion is required for steady-state walking (10° dorsiflexion and 20° plantarflexion) [54,55]. Rotation of the talus within the ankle mortise also occurs and averages 10° [56]. The presence of rotation makes the ankle joint a biplanar articulation. If ankle motion is limited either by disease or an arthrodesis, the second of the three rockers is eliminated. If the sagittal position of the ankle is neutral, the hindfoot and forefoot rockers can compensate for the loss of the second rocker. At heel strike, the Chopart joints plantarflex to promote foot contact with the ground. During midstance, the heel rises earlier, and the weight is transferred more rapidly to the forefoot. Beyaert [57] has demonstrated that the early heel rise and increased anterior tibial tilt during midstance increase the shear forces to the midtarsal joints and are possible reasons for the increased incidence of ipsilateral hindfoot arthritis in patients who have arthritic and stiff ankles or following ankle arthrodesis [58,59].

If the ankle is stiff and in greater than 10° of equinus, a vaulting gait develops with increased knee extension and recurvatum. A patient with an equinus ankle has a slower walking speed and eventually will develop laxity of the medial collateral ligament and posterior capsule of the knee. These abnormalities were not observed in patients whose ankles stiff or fused in a neutral position [60–62]. It also was observed that when the hindfoot was in varus, patients complained of increased pain and callus formation along the lateral border of the foot [60]. If the ankle is painful, the patient adopts an antalgic gait, with a shortened stance phase and insufficient use of the midstance and terminal rocker. This is an energy and a mechanically inefficient gait resulting in significant morbidity [63]. A recent comparative analysis determined that patients who had end-stage ankle arthritis were as disabled as patients who had end-stage hip arthritis.

In the presence of an ankle arthrodesis and a normally functioning subtalar joint complex, the mechanics of gait are affected minimally; there is a slight decrease in stride length and cadence. The oxygen consumption during steady-state walking is increased by 3%, and gait efficiency is 90%. Arthrodesis of the hip has a greater deleterious effect on gait, with oxygen consumption increasing by 32% and gait efficiency decreasing to 53% of normal [64]. With an arthrodesed ankle, walking fast or running is difficult, because the full functional capacity of all three rockers is required during these activities.

The three most important functions of the foot during gait are shock absorption, maintenance of hindfoot stability, and provision of a rocking mechanism. Shock absorption is provided by spring effect of the medial arch and transverse mobility of the subtalar joint complex. Stability is obtained statically by ligament and bony support, and dynamically by the strong lower limb musculature. The rocking mechanism is provided by three components described previously. Ankle stiffness has minimal effect on shock absorption, because most of this is provided by the spring in the medial arch. Ankle arthrodesis allows for maintenance of stability. These are the primary reasons that a stiff painless arthritic ankle in a neutral position does not have the same dramatic deleterious effects on the gait mechanics as knee or hip fusion.

Summary

Normal hindfoot function is imperative for normal gait. The ankle joint plays a pivotal role in imparting stability and flexibility to the hindfoot. Mechanically, the ankle joint is unique in that it accepts the highest load of any joint in the body, with only a third of the contact area as that of the hip and the knee. The thickness of the cartilage mantle is one third of the knee; the cartilage is naturally resilient to the process of aging or degeneration. Stability is imparted by both the ligament and bone (malleoli), and the ankle is the most commonly injured joint in the body. Yet the incidence of arthritis of the ankle joint remains lower than that of the hip or the knee. Physicians have come to understand in greater depth the mechanics of the ankle joint and the function of its cartilage. The hope is that this knowledge eventually will lead to improved treatment options for ankle arthritis.

References

[1] MacConaill M, Basmajian J. Muscles and movements: a basis for human kinesiology. In: MacConaill M, Basmajianed J, editors. Baltimore (MD): The Williams & Wilkins Co; 1969. p. 49.

[2] Cushnaghan J, Dieppe P. Study of 500 patients with limb joint osteoarthritis. I. Analysis by age, sex, and distribution of symptomatic joint sites. Ann Rheum Dis 1991;50:8–13.

[3] Hintermann B, Valderrabano V, Dereymaeker G, et al. The HINTEGRA ankle: rationale and short-term results of 122 consecutive ankles. Clin Orthop Relat Res 2004;(424): 57–68.

[4] Wilson M, Michet CJ Jr, Ilstrup DM, et al. Idiopathic symptomatic osteoarthritis of the hip and knee: a population-based incidence study. Mayo Clin Proc 1990;65:1214–21.

[5] Stauffer R, Chae E, Brewster R. Force and motion analysis of the normal, diseased, and prosthetic ankle joint. Clin Orthop Relat Res 1977;127:189–96.

[6] Agel J, Coetzee JC, Sangeorzan BJ, et al. Functional limitations of patients with end-stage ankle arthrosis. Foot Ankle Int 2005;26(7):537–9.

[7] Wagner FW Jr. Ankle fusion for degenerative arthritis secondary to the collagen diseases. Foot Ankle 1982;3(1):24–31.

[8] Thompson FM, Mann RA. Arthritides. In: Mann RA, Coughlin MJ, editors. Surgery of the foot and ankle. vol. 1. 6th edition. St Louis (MO): Mosby; 1993. p. 664–6.

[9] Harrington KD. Degenerative arthritis of the ankle secondary to long-standing lateral ligament instability. J Bone Joint Surg Am 1979;61(3):354–61.

[10] Lindsjo U. Operative treatment of ankle fracture dislocations. A follow-up study of 306/321 consecutive cases. Clin Orthop 1985;(199):28–38.

[11] Weber BG. [Fractures of the ankle joint and the astragalus. New aspects in diagnosis and treatment (author's translation)]. Langenbecks Arch Chir 1981;355:421–5 [in German].

[12] McDaniel WJ, Wilson FC. Trimalleolar fractures of the ankle. An end result study. Clin Orthop 1977;(122):37–45.

[13] Cedell CA. Supination–outward rotation injuries of the ankle. A clinical and roentgenological study with special reference to the operative treatment. Acta Orthop Scand 1967;(Suppl 110):3, +.

[14] Ruedi T. Fractures of the lower end of the tibia into the ankle joint: results 9 years after open reduction and internal fixation. Injury 1973;5(2):130–4.

[15] Marsh JL, Buckwalter J, Gelberman R, et al. Articular fractures: does an anatomic reduction really change the result? J Bone Joint Surg Am 2002;84(7):1259–71.

[16] Marsh JL, et al. Tibial plafond fractures: does articular reduction and/or injury pattern predict outcome? J Bone Joint Surg Am 2002;84-A(7):1259–71.

[17] Daniels TR, Smith JW. Talar neck fractures. Foot Ankle 1993;14(4):225–34.

[18] Sanders R. Fractures and fracture–dislocations of the talus. In: Coughlin MJ, Mann RA, editors. Surgery of the foot and ankle. vol. 2. 7th edition. St Loius (MO): Mosby Inc; 1999. p. 1465–518.

[19] Treppo S, Koepp H, Quan EC, et al. Comparison of biomechanical and biochemical properties of cartilage from human knee and ankle pairs. J Orthop Res 2000;18(5):739–48.

[20] Shepherd DE, Seedhom BB. Thickness of human articular cartilage in joints of the lower limb. Ann Rheum Dis 1999;58(1):27–34.

[21] Adam C, Eckstein F, Milz S, et al. The distribution of cartilage thickness within the joints of the lower limb of elderly individuals. J Anat 1998;193(Pt 2):203–14.

[22] Simon WH, Friedenberg S, Richardson S. Joint congruence. A correlation of joint congruence and thickness of articular cartilage in dogs. J Bone Joint Surg Am 1973;55(8):1614–20.

[23] Wynarsky GT, Greenwald AS. Mathematical model of the human ankle joint. J Biomech 1983;16(4):241–51.

[24] Wan L, de Asla RJ, Rubash HE, et al. Determination of in vivo articular cartilage contact areas of human talocrural joint under weight-bearing conditions. Osteoarthritis Cartilage 2006;14(12):1294–301.

[25] Brown TD, Shaw DT. In vitro contact stress distributions in the natural human hip. J Biomech 1983;16(6):373–84.

[26] Ihn JC, Kim SJ, Park IH. In vitro study of contact area and pressure distribution in the human knee after partial and total meniscectomy. Int Orthop 1993;17(4):214–8.

[27] Kimizuka M, Kurosawa H, Fukubayashi T. Load-bearing pattern of the ankle joint: contact area and pressure distribution. Arch Orthop Trauma Surg 1980;96:45–9.

[28] Ramsey PL, Hamilton W. Changes in tibio–talar area of contact caused by lateral talar shift. J Bone Joint Surg Am 1976;58(3):356–7.

[29] Lloyd J, Elsayed S, Hariharan K, et al. Revisiting the concept of talar shift in ankle fractures. Foot Ankle Int 2006;27(10):793–6.

[30] Moody M, Koeneman J, Hettinger E, et al. The effects of fibular and talar displacement on joint contact areas about the ankle. Orthop Rev 1992;21(6):741–4.

[31] Clarke HJ, Michelson JD, Cox QG, et al. Tibio–talar stability in bimalleolar ankle fractures: a dynamic in vitro contact area study. Foot Ankle 1991;11(4):222–7.

[32] Pereira DS, Koval KJ, Resnick RB, et al. Tibio talar contact area and pressure distribution: the effect of mortise widening and syndesmosis fixation. Foot Ankle Int 1996;17(5):269–74.

[33] Curtis MJ, Michelson JD, Urquhart MW, et al. Tibio talar contact and fibular malunion in ankle fractures. A cadaver study. Acta Orthop Scand 1992;63(3):326–9.

[34] Kempson GE. Age-related changes in the tensile properties of human articular cartilage: a comparative study between the femoral head of the hip joint and the talus of the ankle joint. Biochim Biophys Acta 1991;1075(3):223–30.

[35] Swann AC, Seedhom BB. The stiffness of normal articular cartilage and the predominant acting stress levels: implications for the aetiology of osteoarthrosis. Br J Rheumatol 1993;32(1):16–25.

[36] Athanasiou KA, Niederauer GG, Schenck RC Jr. Biomechanical topography of human ankle cartilage. Ann Biomed Eng 1995;23(5):697–704.

[37] Palmoski MJ, Brandt KD. Effects of static and cyclic compressive loading on articular cartilage plugs in vitro. Arthritis Rheum 1984;27(6):675–81.

[38] Ins A, et al. Bone density of the human talus does not vary as a function of the cartilage score. Transactions of the Orthopaedic Research Society 1998;23:722.

[39] Cole AA, Chubinskaya S, Schumacher B, et al. Chondrocyte matrix metalloproteinase-8. Human articular chondrocytes express neutrophil collagenase. J Biol Chem 1996;271(18): 11023–6.

[40] Huch K, et al. Human osteoarthritic chondrocytes express message for neutrophil collagenase and stromelysin. Transactions of the Orthopaedic Research Society 1995;20:338.

[41] Chubinskaya S, Huch K, Mikecz K, et al. Chondrocyte matrix metalloproteinase-8: up-regulation of neutrophil collagenase by interleukin-1 beta in human cartilage from knee and ankle joints. Lab Invest 1996;74(1):232–40.

[42] Chubinskaya S, Kuettner KE, Cole AA. Expression of matrix metalloproteinases in normal and damaged articular cartilage from human knee and ankle joints. Lab Invest 1999;79(12): 1669–77.

[43] Kang Y, Koepp H, Cole AA, et al. Cultured human ankle and knee cartilage differ in susceptibility to damage mediated by fibronectin fragments. J Orthop Res 1998;16(5):551–6.

[44] Hauselmann HJ, Mok SS, Flechtenmacher J. Chondrocytes from human knee and ankle joints show differences in responses to IL-1 receptor inhibitor. Transactions of the Orthopaedic Research Society 1993;18:280.

[45] Unsworth A. Tribology of human and artificial joints. Proc Inst Mech Eng [H] 1991;205(3): 163–72.

[46] Huch K, Kuettner KE, Dieppe P. Osteoarthritis in ankle and knee joints. Semin Arthritis Rheum 1997;26(4):667–74.

[47] Koepp H, Eger W, Muehleman C, et al. Prevalence of articular cartilage degeneration in the ankle and knee joints of human organ donors. J Orthop Sci 1999;4(6):407–12.

[48] Meachim G, Emery IH. Quantitative aspects of patello-femoral cartilage fibrillation in Liverpool necropsies. Ann Rheum Dis 1974;33(1):39–47.

[49] Meachim G. Cartilage fibrillation at the ankle joint in Liverpool necropsies. J Anat 1975; 119(3):601–10.

[50] Tsukahara T. [Degeneration of articular cartilage of the ankle in cadavers studied by gross and radiographic examinations]. Nippon Seikeigeka Gakkai Zasshi 1990;64(12):1195–201 [in Japanese].

[51] Muehleman C, Bareither D, Huch K, et al. Prevalence of degenerative morphological changes in the joints of the lower extremity. Osteoarthritis Cartilage 1997;5(1):23–37.

[52] Lynch A, Bourne R, Rorabeck C. The long-term results of ankle arthrodesis. J Bone Joint Surg Am 1988;70:113–6.

[53] Harris GF, Wertsch JJ. Procedures for gait analysis. Arch Phys Med Rehabil 1994;75(2): 216–25.

[54] Kadaba MP, Ramakrishnan HK, Wootten ME, et al. Repeatability of kinematic, kinetic, and electromyographic data in normal adult gait. J Orthop Res 1989;7(6):849–60.

[55] Calhoun JH, Li F, Ledbetter BR, et al. A comprehensive study of pressure distribution in the ankle joint with inversion and eversion. Foot Ankle Int 1994;15(3):125–33.

[56] Lundberg A. Kinematics of the ankle and foot. In vivo roentgen stereophotogrammetry. Acta Orthop Scand Suppl 1989;233:1–24.

[57] Beyaert C, Sirveaux F, Paysant J, et al. The effect of tibio-talar arthrodesis on foot kinematics and ground reaction force progression during walking. Gait Posture 2004;20(1):84–91.

[58] Coester LM, Saltzman CL, Leupold J, et al. Long-term results following ankle arthrodesis for post-traumatic arthritis. J Bone Joint Surg Am 2001;83(2):219–28.

[59] Fuchs S, Sandmann C, Skwara A, et al. Quality of life 20 years after arthrodesis of the ankle. A study of adjacent joints. J Bone Joint Surg Br 2003;85(7):994–8.

[60] Buck P, Morrey B, Chao E. The optimum position of arthrodesis of the ankle. A gait study of the knee and ankle. J Bone Joint Surg Am 1987;69:1052–62.

[61] King HA, Watkins TB Jr, Samuelson KM. Analysis of foot position in ankle arthrodesis and its influence on gait. Foot Ankle 1980;1(1):44–9.

[62] Hefti FL, Baumann JU, Morscher EW. Ankle joint fusion—determination of optimal position by gait analysis. Arch Orthop Trauma Surg 1980;96(3):187–95.

[63] Glazebrook M, Daniels T, Younger A, et al. Comparison of health-related quality of life between patients with end-stage ankle and hip arthrosis. J Bone Joint Surg Am 2008; 90(3):499–505.

[64] Waters RL, Barnes G, Husserl T, et al. Comparable energy expenditure after arthrodesis of the hip and ankle. J Bone Joint Surg Am 1988;70(7):1032–7.

ELSEVIER
SAUNDERS

Foot Ankle Clin N Am
13 (2008) 353–361

FOOT AND
ANKLE CLINICS

Dietary and Viscosupplementation in Ankle Arthritis

Shaun K. Khosla, MD[a], Judith F. Baumhauer, MD[b],*

[a]Department of Orthopaedics, University of Rochester Medical Center, 601 Elmwood Avenue,
Box 665, Rochester, New York 14642, USA
[b]Department of Orthopaedics, Division of Foot and Ankle Surgery, University of Rochester
Medical Center, 601 Elmwood Avenue, Box 665, Rochester, New York 14642, USA

Osteoarthritis is a major debilitating process, causing pain and diminished quality of life. Over the past decades, there have been several orthopaedic developments directed toward pain and functional improvements for people suffering from this most common form of arthritis. These improvements have come in the form of medical management, advanced surgical procedures, joint arthroplasties, and rehabilitation, among others. In the category of medical management, there has been a growing interest in dietary supplementation and viscosupplementation. Most of the past literature regarding these topics has been targeted toward the knee joint; however, more recent publications have investigated these applications in other joints, including the ankle. This article attempts to consolidate these findings and explore the impact of dietary and viscosupplementation in the ankle joint.

Dietary supplementation

A multitude of dietary supplements are on the market, and each year billions of dollars are spent on these supplements and other nutraceuticals by consumers in hopes of improving their health or curing some disease. It is unfortunate that there is little regulation of these compounds. According to the National Institutes of Health [1], "for a new dietary ingredient the manufacturer must notify [the Food and Drug Administration] FDA of its intent to market a dietary supplement containing the new dietary ingredient and provide information on how it determined that reasonable

---

Dr. Baumhauer is a paid consultant for Carticept, Inc., Zimmer and DePuy.
* Corresponding author.
E-mail address: judy_baumhuaer@urmc.rochester.edu (J.F. Baumhauer).

evidence exists for safe human use of the product.... Manufacturers do not have to provide FDA with evidence that dietary supplements are effective or safe; however, they are not permitted to market unsafe or ineffective products. Once a dietary supplement is marketed, FDA has to prove that the product is not safe in order to restrict its use or remove it from the market." In addition, little research data support any of the health claims of many of these products and, as such, their endorsement by the medical community is fairly limited. Due to the increasing public interest in these compounds, however, their existence and claims of health benefits deserve attention. Despite the vast number of supplements on the market, only a subset claims to have an affect on osteoarthritis. Of those, the most heavily marketed and researched are glucosamine and chondroitin sulfate, with their sales alone approaching $730 million in 2004 [2,3].

Glucosamine and chondroitin sulfate

In Europe, glucosamine is marketed as a drug and held to regulatory standards; however, glucosamine and chondroitin sulfate are currently marketed as nutritional supplements in the United States and Canada [4]. Their advertised benefit is aid in relieving symptoms associated with osteoarthritis. To understand their purported effect, one needs to understand their structural and functional role in articular cartilage.

Articular cartilage is composed of chondrocytes within an extracellular matrix. The matrix, in turn, is composed of water, collagens, proteoglycans, and noncollagenous proteins. The frictionless movement and lubrication system of the joint is due in large part to the properties of the extracellular matrix [5]. The proteoglycans in the matrix are made up of glycosaminoglycans and oligosaccharides that, when attached to a protein core, serve as a framework for collagen. The glycosaminoglycans that are most common in cartilage include keratin sulfate, dermatan sulfate, heparin sulfate, and chondroitin sulfate. Glucosamine (2-amino-2-deoxy-α-D-glucose) is an aminosaccharide believed to act as a substrate for the formation of chondroitin sulfate and hyaluronic acid. The chondroitin sulfate chains are a component of aggrecans, one of the larger proteoglycans involved in forming proteoglycan aggregates. The chains are involved in drawing water into the matrix, which significantly contributes to the load-bearing properties of articular cartilage [6–9].

Glucosamine is thought to have its effects by inhibiting the production of interleukin-1-stimulated, proinflammatory mediators such as prostaglandin E2, nitric oxide, NFκβ, and matrix metalloproteinase 1 [10]. One other possibility is that glucosamine may increase production of hyaluronic acid [11]. Chondroitin sulfate may also have a variety of effects, including inhibition of leukocyte elastase, tissue elastase, and the migration of polymorphonuclear leukocytes. Chondroitin sulfate also may increase hyaluronic acid production [12–14].

A number of published studies have examined the effects of glucosamine and chondroitin sulfate in the arthritic population; however, these are primarily limited to short-term studies focusing on the knee joint, with few longer-term studies of efficacy. In addition, there is a broad spectrum of clinical outcomes among these trials, making it difficult to ascertain the true effects of these supplements. Studies focus on the structural effects and the symptomatic relief provided by these compounds.

Glucosamine has been theorized to have joint-preserving qualities in patients who have osteoarthritis. One randomized double-blind placebo-controlled trial was performed to examine the long-term effects of glucosamine on the joint structural changes associated with progression of osteoarthritis. In this trial, 212 patients were randomly assigned to receive pharmaceutic-grade glucosamine sulfate (1500 mg) or placebo once daily for 3 years. Weight-bearing anterior-posterior radiographs taken at baseline, at 1 year, and at 3 years were examined for joint-space width of the medial knee compartment. Results demonstrated no average joint-space loss in patients receiving glucosamine. These results were in contrast to a significant decrease in joint space in patients receiving placebo. There was also significant improvement in the Western Ontario University and the McMaster University (WOMAC) pain and physical function subscales in patients taking glucosamine compared with placebo [15].

One prospective double-blind placebo-controlled trial examined the efficacy and safety of chondroitin sulfate dosed at 1 g/d compared with placebo, with the primary outcome being the Lequesne algofunctional index [6]. The Lequesne index decreased in both groups and trended toward improvement increasing over time in the chondroitin sulfate group, although this did not reach statistical significance. The investigators concluded that chondroitin sulfate leads to improvement in patients who have osteoarthritis; however, further research with longer treatment duration and other function measures needs to be completed. These findings were duplicated for glucosamine in another randomized double-blind placebo-controlled trial in 252 outpatients who had knee osteoarthritis [16]. Results demonstrated significant improvement in the Lequesne severity score after 4 weeks of glucosamine sulfate. Glucosamine was dosed at 1500 mg/d and did not significantly differ from placebo in terms of safety or adverse reactions. It was also noted that 2 to 3 weeks of treatment was necessary for glucosamine to begin to show an effect. The investigators' conclusions were that glucosamine selectively improves symptoms of osteoarthritis.

The benefit of glucosamine has been refuted by other publications. One randomized double-blind placebo-controlled trial of 80 patients used a visual analog scale (VAS) for pain in the affected knee as the primary outcome measure. These investigators found no significant difference in this outcome between the glucosamine and the placebo-controlled groups. With the exception of a mild increase in knee flexion, no significant difference was found in other secondary outcomes, including the WOMAC Osteoarthritis Index and the McGill pain questionnaire [17].

In an effort to bring resolution to questions regarding the differing results and scientific quality of previous studies, the National Institutes of Health sponsored the Glucosamine/chondroitin Arthritis Intervention Trial (GAIT) [3]. The GAIT study was a 24-week randomized double-blind placebo- and celecoxib (Celebrex)-controlled multicenter trial performed to evaluate glucosamine hydrochloride, chondroitin sulfate, or the two in combination for safety and efficacy. The primary outcome was defined as a 20% decrease of the WOMAC pain subscale score. Results showed that the use of glucosamine hydrochloride and chondroitin sulfate, alone or in combination, was not significant with regard to the primary outcome. In the subset of patients who had moderate to severe knee pain, however, combination therapy significantly decreased knee pain as seen in the primary outcome measure. The investigators concluded that combination therapy may be effective in this specific subgroup of arthritis patients.

More recently, the Glucosamine Unum In Die (once-a-day) Efficacy (GUIDE) trial was completed in Europe to assess the effect of glucosamine sulfate on the Lequesne index over a 6-month follow-up period [18]. This study was an industry-sponsored randomized double-blind placebo-controlled trial using acetaminophen as a side comparator. The investigators showed that glucosamine sulfate was significantly more effective than placebo in improving the Lequesne index (3.1 points for glucosamine sulfate versus 1.9 points for placebo).

Differences in the results of these two trials contribute to the controversy regarding the efficacy of these two compounds. Reginster and colleagues [4] stated a number of reasons for the difficulty in interpreting these studies: (1) lack of regulation of the chemical composition of these substance in the United States versus stricter regulation in Europe, (2) possible differing efficacies of glucosamine hydrochloride versus glucosamine sulfate, and (3) higher placebo responses in the GAIT trial versus more average placebo responses in the GUIDE trial.

In light of the varying results of different trials, it is difficult to draw firm conclusions regarding the efficacy of these two compounds. They may provide symptomatic relief in patients who have knee arthritis, especially those who have moderate to severe disease manifestations [3]. In addition, they have few adverse side effects, mainly gastrointestinal discomfort [19]. The most comprehensive analysis comes from the Cochrane Review [20], which included 20 studies and 2570 patients. The conclusions were that WOMAC outcomes of pain and functional impairment did not show a superiority of glucosamine over placebo for the pharmaceutical and the non-pharmaceutical preparations. Further research is needed to determine the ability of glucosamine to relieve symptoms and to delay radiologic progression of osteoarthritis. The Cochrane Review also concluded that glucosamine is as safe as placebo [20]. Again, no data in the literature are specifically directed at symptoms of ankle arthritis; therefore, one can only extrapolate possible effects from studies involving the knee.

Other dietary supplements that are marketed toward relieving osteoarthritic symptoms include S-adenosylmethionine (SAM-e), ginger, dimethyl sulfoxide, and avocado/soybean unsoponifiables [19]. Of these, perhaps the most well-marketed is SAM-e. SAM-e is a sulfur-containing compound made from amino acids that has been reported to decrease pain and joint stiffness in osteoarthritic patients. It is currently available by prescription in Europe [19]. One recent meta-analysis of the literature concluded that SAM-e appears to improve pain and functional limitations coincident with osteoarthritis; however, long-term randomized controlled trials have not investigated these findings [21].

Viscosupplementation

Another nonoperative measure of treating symptoms associated with arthritis is through viscosupplementation by means of hyaluronic acid injections into the affected joint. Hyaluronic acid is a polysaccharide composed of N-acetylglucosamine and glucuronic acid. It is synthesized by type B synoviocytes and secreted into the joint. A nonarthritic knee contains approximately 2.5 to 4.0 mg/mL of high-molecular-weight (5×10^6 d) hyaluronic acid in approximately 2 mL of synovial fluid [5,22]. In an osteoarthritic knee, hyaluronic acid is present in less than half its normal concentration and has altered viscous and elastic properties. There is diminished interaction between the molecules, resulting in reduced barrier and filter effects, which in turn alters stress forces on the articular cartilage and changes in nutrition and waste removal [22].

The thought that viscosupplementation exerts its effect through simple mechanical supplementation of the hyaluronic acid in the joint does not correlate with the fact that the benefits of injection are experienced long after the hyaluronic supplementation is gone from the joint. There have been many other proposed pathways through which hyaluronic acid exerts its effects in osteoarthritic knees. Watterson and Esdaile [22] summarized these mechanisms into anti-inflammatory effects, anabolic effects, and analgesic activity. In terms of anti-inflammatory effects, hyaluronic acid has been shown to inhibit phagocytosis and adherence and to decrease the levels of inflammatory mediators in the synovial fluid of patients who have osteoarthritis [5,22–24]. Intra-articular injections have also been shown to stimulate de novo production of hyaluronic acid, exerting an anabolic effect in osteoarthritic joints. The magnitude of the effect has been linked to the molecular weight of the hyaluronic acid, with a weight of greater than 5×10^5 d most effective [22,25]. Viscosupplementation has also been theorized to enhance cartilage function after injury and to promote chondrocyte proliferation, thereby enhancing the overall integrity of cartilage [26].

The potential analgesic effects are perhaps the main reason for the rising popularity of hyaluronic acid injections in the osteoarthritic population. Hyaluronic acid is currently marketed in the United States for the primary indication of pain [27]. Viscosupplementation for knee arthritis has been in use in the United States since 1997. Hylan G-F 20 (Synvisc) and sodium hyaluronate (Hyalgan) were approved for use by the FDA in 1997, with sodium hyaluronate (Supartz), high-molecular-weight hyaluronan (Orthovisc), and 1% sodium hyaluronate (Euflexxa) soon following suit. It should be noted that these substances are approved for use as a medical device by the FDA, not as a drug.

There have been many studies investigating the effects of viscosupplementation in knee arthritis, the only joint for which it is currently FDA approved. One recent prospective randomized double-blind placebo-controlled trial of 106 patients demonstrated a significant improvement in the WOMAC score and the VAS score compared with the placebo group [28]. These investigators also noted that prolongation of treatment beyond 3 weeks did not appear to make a difference in outcome. The benefit of hyaluronic acid was also shown in an analysis of five double-blind randomized controlled trials that demonstrated a statistically significant reduction in total Lequesne score with hyaluronan versus placebo [29].

As with dietary supplements, there have been some differing results in the literature with regard to the efficacy of hyaluronic acid. One meta-analysis was performed with the goal of determining the therapeutic efficacy and safety, with the hope of reaching a conclusion on the matter [30]. In this meta-analysis of 20 blinded, randomized controlled trials, results showed that cross-linked and non–cross-linked hyaluronic acid may significantly decrease symptoms associated with osteoarthritis of the knee. Controversy still remains, however, regarding the efficacy differences between cross-linked and non–cross-linked hyaluronic acids. Subgroup and meta-regression analysis also showed that patients older than 65 years and those who had advanced radiographic signs of osteoarthritis were less likely to realize a benefit from viscosupplementation. In addition, the study addressed questions of the safety profile of viscosupplementation. The investigators noted few adverse events associated with injection of hyaluronic acid. Minor adverse events included mild localized swelling or pain, with a pooled relative risk of 1.19 for all included trials. Only one major adverse event (described as a painful acute local reaction) occurred with injection of cross-linked hyaluronic acid (Synvisc), with a frequency of 0.7%. This rate is lower than other studies of Synvisc, which cited rates of 2% to 8%. Another article reported the incidence of local reactions after injection of hyaluronic acid to be between 2% and 3%, with symptoms usually resolving within 2 days after administration [26].

One prospective randomized trial of 100 patients compared hyaluronic acid to corticosteroid in terms of symptomatic relief [31]. Hylan G-F 20 was compared with sodium phosphate-betamethasone acetate (Celestone) with regard to WOMAC, the modified Knee Society rating system, and a VAS score. The investigators concluded that the corticosteroid group and the Hylan G-F 20 group demonstrated improvements from baseline;

however, there were no significant differences detected between the two groups.

No viscosupplements have been approved for use in joints other than the knee. That being said, there are preliminary studies being performed to examine the effects of viscosupplementation in other joints commonly affected by osteoarthritis, such as the hip, shoulder, and ankle [32–34]. One study by Sun and colleagues [34] evaluated the effects of viscosupplementation in Kellgren-Lawrence grade I and II ankles. This prospective study included 93 patients who had unilateral ankle pain and were given five weekly injections of sodium hyaluronate (Artz). At the conclusion of the study, the investigators noted a significant decrease in the pain subscale score of the Ankle Osteoarthritis Scale (AOS) and a significant improvement in the American Orthopaedic Foot and Ankle clinical rating scale for the ankle. These changes remained significant at 6 months following the last injection. This study was not blinded and was without a placebo control group; however, the results suggest a benefit for viscosupplementation use in ankle arthritis.

Additional investigations of sodium hyaluronate (Hyalgan) injections in the ankle have yielded similar results. Salk and colleagues [35,36] investigated 20 patients in a randomized double-blind study comparing sodium hyaluronate to a phosphate-buffered saline control. The primary outcome measurement was the AOS score. At 6 months, a decrease in pain and disability as measured by the AOS score was observed, with a trend toward greater improvement in the hyaluronate group. No serious adverse events occurred. Although the study population was small, the results remain suggestive of a beneficial effect of viscosupplementation in ankle arthritis. Studies examining viscosupplementation in the ankle joint are few; however, results seem promising.

Summary

In summary, data regarding dietary supplementation and viscosupplementation and their effects in the ankle joint are still evolving. Glucosamine and chondroitin sulfate are, by far, the most well-marketed dietary supplements directed toward managing symptoms associated with osteoarthritis. The presumption of their benefit in the ankle is based largely on promising results from their use in knee osteoarthritis. Likewise, viscosupplementation has proved to be efficacious in the management of osteoarthritis of the knee. Preliminary studies demonstrate a realization of this benefit in the ankle joint, but further research is required. So far, the literature has shown the dietary and viscosupplementation discussed in this article to be relatively safe for use. Further research should be directed toward randomized double-blind placebo-controlled trials of larger patient populations with established outcome measures. Longer follow-up is also needed to determine the onset and duration of efficacy.

References

[1] Dietary supplements: background information. Office of dietary supplements; National Institutes of Health; 2003.

[2] Annual nutrition industry overview. Nutrition Business Journal 2005;6–7.

[3] Clegg DO, Reda DJ, Harris CL, et al. Glucosamine, chondroitin sulfate, and the two in combination for painful knee osteoarthritis. N Engl J Med 2006;354(8):795–808.

[4] Reginster JY, Bruyere O, Neuprez A. Current role of glucosamine in the treatment of osteoarthritis. Rheumatology 2007;46(5):731–5.

[5] Mankin HJ, Grodzinsky AJ, Buckwalter JA. Articular cartilage and osteoarthritis. In: Einhorn TA, O'Keefe RJ, Buckwalter JA, editors. Orthopaedic basic science: foundations of clinical practice. 3rd edition. Rosemont, IL: American academy of orthopaedic surgeons; 2007. p. 161–74, 329.

[6] Mazieres B, Combe B, Van AP, et al. Chondroitin sulfate in osteoarthritis of the knee: a prospective, double blind, placebo controlled multicenter clinical study. J Rheumatol 2000; 28(1):173–81.

[7] Hungerford DS, Jones LC. Glucosamine and chondroitin sulfate are effective in the management of osteoarthritis. J Arthroplasty 2003;18(3):5–9.

[8] Morris CD. Orthopaedic pharmacology and therapeutics. In: Einhorn TA, O'Keefe RJ, Buckwalter JA, editors. Orthopaedic basic science: foundations of clinical practice. 3rd edition. American academy of orthopaedic surgeons; 2007. p. 329.

[9] Brief AA, Maure SG, Di Cesare PE. Use of glucosamine and chondroitin sulfate in the management of osteoarthritis. J Am Acad Orthop Surg 2001;9(2):71–8.

[10] Alvarez-Soria MA, Largo R, Calvo E, et al. Differential anticatabolic profile of glucosamine sulfate versus other anti-osteoarthritic drugs on human osteoarthritic chondrocytes and synovial fibrolast in culture. Osteoarthritis Cartilage 2005;13:S153.

[11] McCarty MF. Enhanced synovial production of hyaluronic acid may explain rapid clinical response to high-dose glucosamine in osteoarthritis. Med Hypotheses 1998;50:507–10.

[12] Baici A, Bradamante P. Interaction between human leukocyte elastase and chondroitin sulfate. Chem Biol Interact 1984;51:1–11.

[13] Conte A, Pertrini M, Vaglini F, et al. Einige biochemishe mechanismen der entzündungshemmenden aktivität von exognenm chondroiteinsulfat. Letera Rheumatologica 1992;14: 35–42.

[14] Kato Y, Mukudai Y, Okimura A, et al. Effects of hyaluronic acid on the release of cartilage matrix proteoglycan and fibronectin from the cell matrix layer of chondrocyte cultures: interaction between hyaluronic acid and chondroitin sulphate glycosaminoglycan. J Rheumatol 1995;22(Suppl 43):158–9.

[15] Reginster JY, Deroisy R, Rovati LC, et al. Long-term effects of glucosamine sulphate on osteoarthritis progression: a randomized, placebo-controlled clinical trial. Lancet 2001; 357:251–6.

[16] Noack W, Fischer M, Förster KK, et al. Glucosamine sulfate in osteoarthritis of the knee. Osteoarthritis Cartilage 1994;2:51–9.

[17] Hughes R, Carr A. A randomized, double-blind, placebo-controlled trial of glucosamine sulphate as an analgesic in osteoarthritis of the knee. Rheumatology 2002;41:279–84.

[18] Herrero-Beaumont G, Ivorra JAR, Trabado M, et al. Glucosamine sulfate in the treatment of knee osteoarthritis symptoms. Arthritis Rheum 2007;56(2):555–67.

[19] Morelli V, Naquin C, Weaver V. Alternative therapies for traditional disease states: osteoarthritis. Am Fam Physician 2003;67(2):331–44.

[20] Towheed TE, Maxwell L, Anastassiades TP, et al. Glucosamine therapy for treating osteoarthritis. Cochrane Review 2007;4:1–56.

[21] Soeken KL, Lee W, Bausell RB. Safety and efficacy of S-adenosylmethionine for osteoarthritis. J Fam Pract 2002;51(5):425–30.

[22] Watterson JR, Esdaile JM. Viscosupplementation: therapeutic mechanisms and clinical potential in osteoarthritis of the knee. J Am Acad Orthop Surg 2000;8:277–84.

[23] Forrester JV, Balazs EA. Inhibition of phagocytosis by high molecular weight hyaluronate. Immunology 1980;40:435–46.

[24] Stitik TP, Levy JA. Viscosupplementation for osteoarthritis. Am J Phys Med Rehabil 2006; 85(Suppl):S32–50.

[25] Smith MM, Ghosh P. The synthesis of hyaluronic acid by human synovial fibroblasts is influenced by the nature of the hyaluronate in the extracellular environment. Rheumatol Int 1987;(7):113–22.

[26] Marshall KW. Intra-articular hyaluronan therapy. Foot Ankle Clin N Am 2003;8:221–32.

[27] Prescriber Information, Hyalgan, Sanofi Aventis. New York; July, 2001.

[28] Petrella RJ, Petrella M. A prospective, randomized, double-blind, placebo controlled study to evaluate the efficacy of intraarticular hyaluronic acid for osteoarthritis of the knee. J Rheumatol 2006;33(5):951–6.

[29] Strand V, Conaghan PG, Lohmander LS. An integrated analysis of five double-blind, randomized controlled trials evaluating the safety and efficacy of a hyaluronan product for intra-articular injection in osteoarthritis of the knee. Osteoarthritis Cartilage 2006;14: 859–66.

[30] Wang CT, Lin J, Chang CJ. Therapeautic effects of hyaluronic acid on osteoarthritis of the knee. J Bone Joint Surg Am 2004;86:538–45.

[31] Leopold SS, Redd BB, Warme WJ. Corticosteroid compared with hyaluronic acid injections for the treatment of osteoarthritis of the knee. J Bone Joint Surg AM 2003;85(7):1197–203.

[32] Lopez JCF, Ruano-Ravina A. Efficacy and safety of intraarticular hyaluronic acid the treatment of hip osteoarthritis: a systematic review. Osteoarthritis Cartilage 2006;14:1306–11.

[33] Silverstein E, Leger R, Shea KP. The use of intra-articular Hylan G-F 20 in the treatment of symptomatic osteoarthritis of the shoulder. Am J Sports Med 2007;35:979–86.

[34] Sun SF, Chou YJ, Hsu CW, et al. Efficacy of intra-articular hyaluronic acid in patients with osteoarthritis of the ankle: a prospective study. Osteoarthritis Cartilage 2006;14:867–74.

[35] Salk RS, Chang TJ, D'Costa WF, et al. Sodium hyaluronate in the treatment of osteoarthritis of the ankle: a controlled, randomized double-blind pilot study. J Bone Joint Surg AM 2006;88(2):295–302.

[36] Salk R, Chang T, D'Costa W, et al. Viscosupplementation in the treatment of ankle osteoarthritis. Clin Podiatr Med Surg 2005;22:585–97.

ELSEVIER
SAUNDERS

Foot Ankle Clin N Am
13 (2008) 363–379

FOOT AND
ANKLE CLINICS

Stimulation of Ankle Cartilage: Other Emerging Technologies (Cellular, Electricomagnetic, etc.)

Tamir Bloom, MD[a],*, Regis Renard, MD[b],
Praveen Yalamanchili, MD[b], Keith Wapner, MD[c],
Wen Chao, MD[c], Sheldon S. Lin, MD[d]

[a]Division of Pediatric Othopaedics, Department of Orthopaedic Surgery, New Jersey Medical
School—University of Medicine and Dentistry of New Jersey,
90 Bergen Street, Suite 1200, Newark, NJ 07103, USA
[b]Department of Orthopaedic Surgery, New Jersey Medical School—University of Medicine
and Dentistry of New Jersey, 90 Bergen Street, Suite 1200, Newark, NJ 07103, USA
[c]Department of Orthopaedic Surgery, University of Pennsylvania, USA
[d]Foot and Ankle Division, Department of Orthopaedic Surgery, New Jersey Medical
School—University of Medicine and Dentistry of New Jersey,
90 Bergen Street, Suite 1200, Newark, NJ 07103, USA

Orthopedic management of osteoarthritis (OA) of the ankle is based on pain, deformity, instability, functional decline, and the progressive natural history of this degenerative disorder. Despite the overall low incidence of ankle OA compared with the hip and knee, the relatively young average age of presentation of painful ankle OA—the majority of which is associated with previous trauma—is concerning because of the lack of available long-lasting, joint-preserving treatments [1,2]. Ankle arthrodesis remains the gold standard for patients who have diffuse ankle OA and pain after failure of nonsurgical treatment methods. Long-term follow-up, however, demonstrates a significant rate of progressive ipsilateral foot joint arthrosis, overall pain, and functional limitations [3]. Although arthroplasty techniques and implants continue to evolve, arthroplasty is less than ideal for active young and early middle-aged patients because of their limited lifespan.

Surgical "joint sparing" options—including open or arthroscopic débridement, subchondral drilling, realignment osteotomies, osteochondral

---

* Corresponding author.
E-mail address: bloomta@umdnj.edu (T. Bloom).

shell allograft reconstruction, and distraction osteogenesis—are more desirable in younger patients. They do not "burn bridges" and allow for arthrodesis or arthroplasty, if needed, at a later time. The indications for these procedures are evolving. Giannini and colleagues [4] recently described their treatment decision-making algorithm based on their management of 190 patients who had posttraumatic ankle OA.

Over the past 2 decades, basic science research in the field of cartilage repair has expanded dramatically. Advances in understanding age-related changes in articular cartilage, joint homeostasis, the natural healing process after cartilage injury, and improved standards for evaluation of a joint surface, made the ultimate goal of cartilage repair a possibility. New strategies for enhancement of articular cartilages' limited healing potential and biologic regeneration include advances in tissue engineering and the use of electromagnetic fields. This article reviews developments in basic science and clinical research made with these emerging technologies concerning treatment of articular cartilage defects and treatment of OA of the ankle.

The role of growth factors in articular cartilage repair

Tissue engineering methods for the biologic repair of articular cartilage involve the development of suitable scaffolds or matrices that can retain and sustain cultured cells and bioactive factors that stimulate extracellular matrix synthesis and regulate ossification. After arthroscopic implantation, biologic matrices augmented with biologic adjuncts (ie, growth factors) are conceptually believed to overcome the limited capacity of cartilage to heal by initiating chondrogenesis, regulating ossification, and improve incorporation to the native cartilage [5]. A variety of biologic adjuncts exists in addition to autograft and allograft bone scaffolds to supplement the surgical treatment of traumatic OA lesions of articular cartilage about the foot and ankle. Current research in this field has tried to understand the role of individual growth factors in cartilage healing, although it is widely believed that ultimately an array of bioactive agents may be required to restore intra-articular cartilage. The most studied growth factors for potential application in cartilage tissue engineering—insulin-like growth factor (IGF), bone morphogenic proteins (BMPs), and platelet-derived growth factor (PDGF)—are discussed.

Insulin-like growth factor

IGF is a single polypeptide with a sequence similar to insulin and has two distinct subtypes, IGF-1 and IGF-2. IGF-1 is an important physiologic mediator and stimulus for growth that is produced mainly in the liver in response to stimulation by growth hormone. Receptors to IGF-1 have been identified in almost all cell types. IGF-1 has been widely studied with respect to cartilage development, homeostasis, and repair [6]. IGF-2 is believed more important in fetal development.

In vitro studies demonstrate a dose-dependent increase in proteoglycan production by chondrocytes in response [7] and concomitant dose-dependent reduction of proteoglycan degradation in response to IGF-1. IGF-1 also may promote the formation of collagen networks via increased proteoglycan and collagen deposition [8]. With age, the decline of chondrocyte synthetic activity in articular cartilage is suggested to be a result of decreased sensitivity to IGF-1, mediated by increased expression of IGF-binding proteins [9]. Arthritic or inflamed articular chondrocytes have a reduced responsiveness to proteoglycan synthesis stimulated by IGF-1, despite chondrocyte up-regulation of IGF-binding proteins, which may indicate receptor function defect in aged or arthritic chondrocytes [7,10–15]. In vitro proteoglycan synthesis from arthritic chondrocytes recovers after stimulation of IGF-1 with the addition of the corticosteroid triamcinolone [7].

Several in vivo studies have demonstrated the effectiveness of IGF-1 in the treatment of cartilage defects in horse, rabbit, and dog models. Nixon and colleagues [16] used their technique for culture and cryopreservation of articular chondrocytes to treat 1.5-cm diameter, full-thickness chondral defects in equine femoral trochlea with fibrin composites with and without the addition of IGF-1 [17]. At 6-months, all animals were sacrificed. The IGF-1–treated group displayed improved tissue fill of the defect, more secure attachment to the subchondral bone, increased amounts of type II collagen, and significantly better histologic healing scores than the controls. Neither group, however, had healed the defects with tissue having biochemical or morphologic features consistent to normal articular cartilage.

In 2002, these investigators reported on the use of a composite of polymerized fibrin and chondrocytes supplemented with IGF-I for arthroscopic repair of full-thickness cartilage defects in horses [18]. At 8 months, repair tissue analysis of postmortem specimens showed that the addition of IGF-I to chondrocyte grafts enhanced chondrogenesis in cartilage defects, including graft incorporation. In addition, gross filling of defects was improved, and the tissue contained a higher proportion of cells producing type II collagen.

Recently, Goodrich and colleagues [19] arthroscopically grafted chondrocytes genetically modified by an adenovirus vector-encoding equine IGF-1 (AdIGF-1) in an equine femoropatellar joint model. A single 15-mm cartilage full-thickness defect was created in each femoropatellar joint in 16 horses. One joint received vector-modified chondrocytes (AdIGF-1), and the contralateral side received unmodified chondrocytes. In defects treated with the modified chondrocytes, gross and histologic appearance improved, with increased defect filling with hyaline cartilage.

In a rabbit model, Madry and colleagues [20] successfully used plasmid vectors to transfect chondrocytes to overexpress the IGF-I gene and then transplanted into osteochondral defects in the trochlear groove. At 3 and 14 weeks, transplantation of IGF-I implants secreted biologically relevant amounts of IGF, improved articular cartilage repair, and accelerated the formation of the subchondral. Both studies demonstrated that the trans-fected, allogenic chondrocytes overexpressing IGF-1 increased the expres-sion of type II collagen with improved hyaline-like cartilage repair.

Morisset and colleagues [21] reported on the effect of intra-articular injection of an adenovirus vector of IGF-1 and interleukin (IL)-1 receptor antagonist genes into equine full-thickness, chondral defects treated con-comitantly by arthroscopic, microfracture techniques. At 16 weeks, these in-vestigators noted increased proteoglycan content compared with controls, with augmented type II collagen associated with the gene therapy group. There was no significant improvement, however, in macroscopic and histo-morphometric measurements of the repair tissue between groups.

In a canine model of OA created by transection of the anterior cruciate ligament (ACL), Rogachefsky and colleagues [22] demonstrated that an in-tra-articular injection of IGF-1 combined with an intramusclar injection of sodium pentosan polysulfate (PPS) decreased the progression of articular cartilage degeneration, possibly by decreasing levels of active neutral metal-loproteinases compared with the OA group. They hypothesized PPS inhibited proteinase activity and that this allowed the observed IGF-I–induced effects.

Bone morphogenic protein

BMPs are a group of molecules of the transforming growth factor-beta (TGF-β) superfamily that have a variety of regulatory effects in the differen-tiation of musculoskeletal tissues, including bone and articular cartilage re-pair pathways [23]. Members of this family have been shown to induce bone formation in nonbony sites via endochondral ossification [24,25] and in high concentrations may form bone via intramembranous ossification [26]. BMPs modulate osteoprogenitor and mesenchymal stem cells and are expressed by osteoblasts and chondrocytes. At least 20 types of BMPs have been identi-fied, of which BMP-7 (osteogenic protein 1[OP-1]) has been extensively in-vestigated for its potential in augmentation of cartilage repair [27,28].

In vitro studies indicate that BMP-7 up-regulates chondrocyte metabo-lism and synthesis of cartilage-specific extracellular matrix proteins, includ-ing type II collagen and aggrecan [29–32]. BMP-7 up-regulates expression of a tissue inhibitor of metalloproteinase whereas it inhibits the expression of matrix degradation enzymes and cartilage catabolic mediators [29,33]. BMP-7 promotes the production of normal, functional proteoglycans in normal and OA chondrocytes [32,34,35]. Loeser and colleagues [31] have demonstrated that BMP-7 when combined with IGF-1 has synergistic effects on chondrocyte survival, proliferation, and matrix protein synthesis. Chu-binskaya and colleagues [28] recently published a comprehensive review of the current understanding of BMP-7 as a unique cartilage repair factor, sum-marizing the in vitro and in vivo effects of recombinant human BMP-7 (rhBMP-7).

Early articular cartilage repair studies using BMP-7 were performed in rabbits with bone-derived type I collagen as a graft. Grgic and associates [36] treated full-thickness (3-mm wide) osteochondral defects in rabbit knees with a BMP-7 loaded on a collagen scaffold and noted that the repair tissue contained cells resembling mature chondrocytes compared with controls. Kuo and colleagues [37] reported on treating full-thickness osteochondral defects in rabbit knees by combining microfracture with BMP-7. Defects were made in the patellar grooves of 40 knees and then received (1) no intervention, (2) microfracture, (3) BMP-7, (4) microfracture with BMP-7 in a collagen sponge (combination treatment), or (5) microfracture with a collagen sponge. Animals were sacrificed after 24 weeks at 39 weeks of age. Compared to controls or single treatment, microfracture with the implantation of BMP-7 in a collagen sponge demonstrated a repair response most resembling native hyaline articlar cartilage in quality and quantity of repair tissue. The investigators concluded that microfracture and BMP-7 augmentation act synergistically to enhance cartilage repair.

Mason and colleagues [38] used gene therapy techniques combined with tissue engineering to treat osteochondral defects in rabbit knees. A retroviral vector was used to introduce rhBMP-7 into periosteal-derived rabbit mesenchymal stem cells. These cells were cultured, then seeded onto polyglycolic acid grafts, which were implanted into osteochondral defects model. Defects were harvested after 4, 8, and 12 weeks and evaluated by macroscopic, histologic, and immunohistologic criteria. The grafts containing BMP-7 gene–modified cells consistently showed complete or near complete bone and articular cartilage regeneration at 8 and 12 weeks, whereas the grafts from the control groups had poor repair.

These encouraging results with BMP-7 were followed with experiments in larger animals, including dogs, sheep, and horses. In canine knees, full-thickness osteochondral defects (5-mm diameter by 6-mm deep) treated with rhBMP-7 on a collagen scaffold exhibited improved histologic appearance of repair tissue, resembling mature articular hyaline cartilage compared with controls that had tissue repair of fibrous tissue and fibrocartilage [39]. Recombinant human OP-1–induced repair tissue were maintained at 52 weeks postoperatively.

Focal chondral defects (defects superficial to subchondral bone) also are shown capable of repair in the presence of BMP-7. In a sheep model using an implanted pump to deliver intra-articular rhBMP-7 for 2 weeks after the creation of 10-mm diameter knee chondral lesions, Jelic and associates [40] showed induced defect fill at 3 and 6 months after the surgery. Defects were repaired with regenerate cartilage with high levels of type II collagen as compared with controls who failed to show healing at 3 and 6 months. In an equine model, implantation of genetically modified articular chondrocytes expressing adenovirus vector BMP-7 into 15-mm diameter, full-thickness chondral patellofemoral defects showed an increase in BMP-7 expression with accelerated defect healing [41]. Biopsies at 4 weeks showed repair tissue to have hyaline-like cartilage morphology compared with chondrocytes that did not express BMP-7. By 8 months, however, controls and BMP-7 transfected groups had similar histologic, biochemical, and biomechanical properties.

In addition to its anabolic effects on articular chondrocytes, BMP-7 has anticatabolic effects that may be beneficial for chondroprotection in the setting of OA prevention [28]. In an OA model using ACL-transected rabbit knees, Badlani and colleagues [42] injected BMP-7 continuously for 6 weeks by a catheter from an implantable osmotic pump. At 9 weeks, animals were sacrificed (20 control and 20 experimental). Compared to controls, BMP-7–treated animals showed lower Outerbridge scores, less histomorphologic degeneration, significantly greater expression of aggrecan and collagen type II, and less expression of aggrecanase, suggesting that BMP-7 may be chondroprotective in OA. In a sheep model, BMP-7 prevented posttraumatic OA when two intra-articular injections were administered at the time of injury and 1 week later [43]. These data and studies showing BMP-7 may suppress chondrocyte apoptosis [44] and proteoglygan loss [33,45] suggest that BMP-7 may prevent or delay further chondral damage after injury and possibly stimulate chondrocyte viability and repair.

Platelet-derived growth factor

PDGF is a dimeric glycoprotein consisting of two distinct, disulfide-linked peptide chains (A and B) found as a homodimer (PDGF-AA or PDGF-BB) or as a heterodimer (PDGF-AB). PDGF is produced in smooth-muscle cells and endothelium and stored in high concentrations in platelets. PDGF is an important chemotactic and mitogenic factor in osteoprogenitor cell differentiation toward an osteoblastic lineage [46], secreted by platelets during the early phases of fracture healing [47]. PDGF-receptors are found on many cells, including chondrocytes [48].

In vitro studies on the effects of PDGF on articular chondrocytes seem conflicting. Smith and colleagues [48] demonstated that PDGF-BB in the presence of recombinant human IL-1α resulted in an up-regulation of metalloproteinase and prostaglandin E2 and up-regulated the expression of IL-1α receptors, suggesting that PDGF-BB may be involved in the pathogenesis of arthritic disease with reduction of extracellular matrix. Kieswetter and colleagues [49] examined the effects of PDGF-BB on in vitro cultures of rat resting zone costochodral chondrocytes. PDGF-BB caused a dose-dependent proliferation of chondrocytes and increased proteoglycan production but had no effect on differentiation of cells along the endochondral maturation pathway. Gaissmaier and colleagues [50] studied the in vitro effect of human platelet supernatant (hPS) on human articular chondrocyte cultures. hPS is composed of a milieu of growth factors but rich in PDGF-AB and TGF-β. These investigators demonstrated an enhanced chondrocyte proliferation and, as noted by Kieswetter and coworkers [49], induced chondrocyte dedifferentiation toward a fibroblast-like phenotype. A decrease in expression of mRNAs for type II collagen, aggrecan, and BMP-2 was noted. The investigators concluded that application of hPS would require additional phenotype stabilizing factors to maintain chondrocytes capable of producing hyaline-like cartilage.

Lohmann and colleagues [51] examined the ability of costochondral chondrocytes in a rat model to synthesize cartilage when incorporated into a polylactic/polyglycolic acid scaffold and implanted into mouse calves. Costochondral chondrocytes were pretreated with PDGF-BB at 4 or 24 hours before implantation. The investigators noted a time-dependent decrease of cartilage formation with chondrocytes pretreated 4 hours before implantation producing more cartilage after 8 weeks compared with those pretreated 24 hours before implantation. PDGF-BB decreased the formation of hypertrophic chondrocytes and promoted the retention of hyaline-like chondrogenic phenotype as opposed to endochondral cartilage. These investigators believed that this may be a mechanism to provide heterotopic autogenous cartilage.

Summary of current growth factor use in articular cartilage repair

IGF-1 and BMP-7 increase proteoglycans, type II collagen, and aggrecan and act as an anabolic factor for articular chondrocytes in vitro. BMP-7 is important in cartilage homeostasis and repair. In addition to its anabolic effects, it inhibits cartilage catabolic mediators and degradative enzymes. Both of these growth factors demonstrate the ability to produce hyaline-like cartilage in various types of focal articular cartilage defects and, when used in conjunction with other surgical techniques, such as microfracture, display improved histologic and biochemical aspects of repair tissue (Tables 1 and 2). Furthermore, there is some evidence to support synergistic effects among various biologic adjuncts on cartilage repair. PDGF may have a weak role in the proliferation of chondrocytes for cartilage repair (Table 3).

Future research is required to evaluate formulations, optimal dose, delivery systems, safety profile, and possible combinations of growth factors and elucidate temporal expression of these growth factors on the cartilage microenvironment to optimize cartilage repairs. Current literature on the role of bioactive factors in cartilage repair shows great promise for the future of tissue engineering. Although human trials are not yet in progress, tissue engineering research on articular cartilage repair is entirely concentrated on knee articular cartilage. Extrapolating these results to ankle cartilage may yield different results. The biology and biochemical composition of human articular cartilage in the knee is comparable to the ankle; it is well known that there are significant biomechanical differences and rates of OA [1]. Furthermore, ankle cartilage is shown to differ in matrix composition, water content, and transport properties, all of which effect chondrocyte stimulation response, effective concentration of growth factors, and cytokines to which

Table 1
Effects of insulin-like growth factor 1 on articular cartilage repair

In vitro response	
• Stimulates proteoglycan synthesis	Verschure et al 1994 [7]
• Promotes formation of collagen networks	Jenniskens et al 2006 [8]
In vitro response	
• Hyaline-like repair, with increased type II collagen and more secure subchondral bone attachment in full-thickness chondral defects repaired with fibrin-loaded IGF-1 plugs in equine model	Nixon et al 1992 [16]
• Augmentation of IGF-1 to fibrin-chondrocyte plugs for full-thickness chondral defects in equine model have hyaline-like repair with improved attachment to surrounding cartilage and production type II collagen	Fortier et al 2002 [18]
• Rabbit osteochondral defects repaired with transfected, allogenic chondrocytes overexpressing IGF-1 within an alginate plug had more hyaline-like repair with increased type II collagen expression	Madry et al 2005 [20]
• Increased hyaline-like repair tissue with increased expression of type II collagen was noted in a full-thickness equine chondral defect treated with transfected chondrocytes over expressing IGF-1 added to fibrin plugs	Goodrich et al 2007 [19]
• Intra-articular injections of adenovirus vector of IGF-1 into equine chondral defect knees treated arthroscopically with microfracture had increased production of proteoglycans	Morisset et al 2007 [21]

chondrocytes are exposed and, possibly, underlie the differences in the incidence of OA in these joints [52,53].

The role of electromagnetic techniques in articular cartilage repair

The ability of electromagnetic fields to regulate the gene expression in various connective tissue cells is now well known. Electromagnetic therapy in relation to fracture healing has been studied for decades in the orthopedic literature since the initial observation of electric fields in mechanically loaded bones [54]. There is growing interest in the usefulness of electric fields for articular cartilage preservation and regeneration. Aaron and colleagues [55] illustrated three methods currently in use for applying an electromagnetic field to bone. Invasive methods allow for the use of direct electrical current whereas noninvasive methods use capacitive coupling (CC) or inductive coupling (IC). IC induces a secondary field within the target tissue and can be applied in a series of pulses to create a pulsed electromagnetic field (PEMF). The exact characteristics of the electromagnetic field stimulating the target tissue are determined by a variety of factors, including the applied field and the biologic properties of the tissue.

Table 2
Effects of bone morphogenetic protein 7 on articular cartilage repair

In vitro response	
• Stimulates proteoglycan synthesis in normal and OA chondrocytes	Nishida et al 2000 [32]
• Increases type II collagen synthesis in normal and OA chondrocytes	Chubinskaya et al 2002 [34]
• Stimulates secretion of tissue inhibitor of metalloproteases	Fan et al 2004 [29]
• Inhibits expression of cartilage matrix degradation enzymes and mediators of cartilage catabolism	Nishida et al 2004 [33]
In vivo response	
• Hyaline-like repair, with increased type II collagen and the presence of mature chondrocyte-like cells were observed in rabbit osteochondral defects repaired with BMP-7 loaded collagen plug	Grgic et al 1997 [36]
• Full-thickness chondral defects in rabbit knees treated by microfracture and with a BMP-7 collagen sponge implanted into the defect had improved hyaline-like tissue with increased chondrocyte distribution in the repair tissue	Kuo et al 2006 [37]
• Rabbit osteochondral defects repaired with transfected mesenchymal cells overexpressing BMP-7 within an collagen plug had more hyaline-like repair with increased type II collagen	Mason et al 2000 [38]
• Increased hyaline-like repair tissue with increased expression of type II collagen was noted in canine osteochondral defects treated with BMP-7 loaded collagen plug	Cook et al 2003 [39]
• Full-thickness equine chondral defects treated with transfected chondrocytes overexpressing BMP-7 added to fibrin plugs had accelerated healing with increased hyaline-like repair tissue after 4-months	Hidaka et al 2003 [41]
• Intra-articular BMP-7 injections had chondrocyte protective role in rabbit ACL-transection knees	Badlani et al 2007 [42]
• Intra-articular injections of BMP-7 into sheep chondral defect knees induced fill with increased production of type II collagen	Jelic et al 2001 [40]

Multiple studies exists that aim to elucidate the mechanism of action of electromagnetic fields. On the macroscopic level, one hypothesis is that a mechanical-electric phenomenon exists whereby mechanical compression of cartilage causes stimulation of matrix protein synthesis [56]. At the cellular level, the exact biophysical interaction between electromagnetic fields and cellular membranes is not well established, but membrane-level interactions are an important mediator of downstream effects. A recently proposed theory is that the forced vibration of free ions on the plasma membrane's surface affects the cell's electrochemical balance through irregular gating of electrosensitive channels on the plasma membrane [57]. Another proposed mechanism of action at the cellular membrane is through interaction with various transmembrane receptors. Multiple studies have shown the

Table 3
Effects of platelet-derived growth factor on articular cartilage repair

In vitro response	
• Stimulates proteoglycan synthesis and inhibits chondrocyte maturation	Kieswetter et al 1997 [49]
• Stimulates chondrocyte proliferation and prevents chondrocyte terminal differentiation	Gaissmaier et al 2005 [50]
In vivo response	
• Promotes ectopic cartilage formation with hyaline-like tissue containing immature articular-like chondrocytes	Lohmann et al 2000 [51]

interaction of IC fields with parathyroid hormone receptors [58,59]. Hiraki and colleagues [60] showed increased differentiation of cultured chondrocytes in a rabbit model through PEMF-mediated amplification of response to parathyroid hormone. Other receptors reported effected by electromagnetic fields include insulin, IL-2, IGF-II, transferrin, low-density lipoprotein, calcitonin, and adenosine A_{2A} [61].

Calcium plays an important role as mediator in the action of electromagnetic fields at the cellular level. Various studies have shown an increase in cytosolic calcium concentration after exposure to electromagnetic fields [62,63]. The mechanism of calcium ion translocation, however, seems to vary depending on the type of current used. CC seems to induce calcium ion influx from extracellular matrix via voltage-gated ion channels whereas IC stimulation seems to release intracellular ion stores [61]. The increased amount of intracellular calcium in turn can activate calmodulin, which has a positive effect on cell proliferation.

Electromagnetic fields also seems to stimulate growth factor synthesis. The majority of interest has focused on osteogenesis, where electromagnetic field exposure has been shown to increase mRNA expression of several BMPs and TGF-β [64,65]. Aaron and colleagues [66] studied chondroprogenitor cell differentiation in an enchondral bone ossification model and found that exposure to an electromagnetic field enhanced chondrogenesis TGF-β. In addition, the investigators found a 64% increase in glycosaminoglycan content compared with controls related to increased chondrocyte differentiation. There also were greater levels of aggrecan, type II collagen mRNA, and deposition of proteoglycans.

Many in vitro studies have been published over the past decade that suggest a positive influence on articular hyaline cartilage by electromagnetic fields [56]. Sakai and colleagues [67] found that PEMF stimulation in articular cartilage cells promoted cell proliferation but did not affect glycosaminoglycan production. This effect was most pronounced with intermittent PEMF stimulation. De Mattei and colleagues [68] showed that low-energy, low-frequency PEMFs can induce cell proliferation in human articular chondrocytes, which is sustained longer in low-density chondrocyte cultures than high-density cultures. The investigators suggest that the availability of growth factors and the environmental constrictions affect chondrocyte response to PEMF. Fioravanti and colleagues [69] attempted to evaluate the effect of electromagnetic field therapy in an in vitro OA model by using IL-1. PEMF was able to compensate for IL-1 mediated inhibition of proteoglycan synthesis in human cartilage.

In vivo studies of electromagnetic fields and articular cartilage have focused on Dunkin-Hartley guinea pigs, which develop OA of the knee at 3 months of age and progress to severe OA by 1 year [56]. Ciombor and colleagues [70] described a protective effect of PEMF in this animal model. Subjects exposed to PEMF treatment showed decreased development of OA lesions and increased preservation of tibial plateau articular morphology. There also was a suppression of matrix-degrading enzymes and cells immunopositive to IL-1 and marked increase in the number of cells immunopositive to TGF-β. The investigators suggested that up-regulation of TGF-β may be the mechanism through which PEMF favorably affects cartilage homeostasis. TGF-β has several important regulatory effects in the maintenance of cartilage extracellular matrix morphology, including up-regulation of the gene expression for aggrecan and for inhibitors of matrix metalloprotease and down-regulation of matrix-degrading enzymes and IL-1 activity [71,72]. Fini and colleagues [73] performed a similar study in Dunkin-Hartley guinea pigs and showed that PEMF-treated animals had a significant reduction of chondropathy progression and cartilage thickness was significantly higher in the medial tibia plateaus of the PEMF-treated group than controls. A recent article found that PEMF stimulation could have a chondroprotective effect on OA progression even in severely affected knee joints in elderly guinea pigs [74].

Clinical series of pulsed electromagnetic field treatment

Although many clinical studies exist investigating the use of electromagnetic fields in the treatment of fractures and nonunions, clinical studies studying their use in OA have been fewer and focused mostly regions of the neck and knee. A multicenter randomized controlled trial compared patients who had OA of the knee treated with PEMF and those receiving a placebo. PEMF-treated patients had significantly greater improvement in pain, function, physician global evaluation, and mean morning stiffness over the 4-week treatment time [75]. Another randomized, double-blind clinical trial investigated PEMF in the treatment of OA of the knee and cervical spine [76]. Patients treated with PEMF showed significant improvements from baseline for pain, pain on motion, patient overall assessment, and physician global assessment in contrast to the placebo patients. Pipitone and Scott [77] investigated symptomatic OA of the knee and found that patients treated with PEMF showed significant improvements in a global, pain, and disability score, without any clinically relevant adverse effects. A Cochrane review published in 2002 showed a statistically significant but clinically insignificant benefit of PEMF for treating knee or cervical OA, but the investigators highlighted the paucity of studies available and the need for further large studies before drawing a definitive conclusion [78]. The studies are promising, but it is not possible to determine whether or not the clinical improvements are related simply to symptomatic improvement or to preservation and restoration of cartilage.

An unpublished study looking specifically the benefit of PEMF in talar dome articular cartilage recently was undertaken by Chao and colleagues (Chao W and colleagues, personal communication, 2008). Sixty patients who had microtrabecular fracture of the talus, with or without an osteochondral lesion (Berndt and Harty type I/II), and persistent ankle pain were treated with PEMF bone-stimulating device after failing at least 3 months of protected weight bearing, CAM walker, or casting. The microtrabecular fracture of the talus was diagnosed with MR imaging of the affected ankle. All of the patients had persistent marrow edema in the talus and pain at the location of the marrow edema at the time that the PEMF bone-stimulating device was applied. Patients who had ankle instability were excluded. Failure of PEMF bone-stimulating device was defined as persistent pain after at least of 3 months of usage.

Thirty-three men and 27 women were included in this study. The average age was 39.4 years (range 18–68). Forty-four patients (73.3%) were treated successfully with PEMF bone-stimulating device. In this group of patients, the ankle pain resolved and no further treatment was necessary. Sixteen patients had persistent pain after at least 3 months of using PEMF bone-stimulating device. In this group of patients, all had an osteochondral lesion of the talus. All of the patients in this group underwent arthroscopic debridement and curettage of the osteochondral lesion.

Summary of electromagnetic field therapy in articular cartilage repair

Electromagnetic field therapy is a modality that has been known for decades but recently has come under increased interest as a treatment of OA. The mechanism of action is complex, effecting cell membrane channels and receptors, calcium levels, and the production of cytokines. In vitro and in vivo studies have demonstrated the effectiveness of electromagnetic fields on the proliferation of chondrocytes and the preservation of articular cartilage. Clinical studies, although limited, have demonstrated improvement in pain and function in the setting of knee OA and talar OCD. Whether or not the improvement is purely symptomatic or the result of a chondroprotective effect at the cellular level is unknown. The studies are promising, but it is not possible to determine whether or not the clinical improvements are related simply to symptomatic improvement or to preservation and restoration of cartilage.

Summary

IGF-1 and BMP-7/OP-1 play an important role in stimulating chondrocye differenciation, extracellular matrix production, and preserving mature chondrocytes against the degenerative effects of catabolic mediators. When delivered locally with an appropriate scaffold material, or in some cases intra-articularly through a minipump, these growth factors are demonstrated to improve histologic and biochemical aspects of repair tissue in animal osteochondral and chondral lesions. PDGF may have a role in the proliferation of chondrocytes for cartilage repair. Growth factors, specifically BMP-7, could be used to augment current articular cartilage repair techniques, such as mosaicplasty, microfracture, and cell-based therapies [28]. Future studies are needed to determine the most successful formulations, scaffolds, methods of administration, and possibly combinations with other biologic factors. Evaluation of IGF, BMP, and PDGF for human articular cartilage repair may be expected in the near future.

In vitro and in vivo studies have demonstrated the effectiveness of electromagnetic fields on the proliferation of chondrocytes and the preservation of articular cartilage. Limited clinical studies have demonstrated improvement in pain and function for OA about the knee and ankle. Whether or not this modality holds significant theraputic promise in cartilage repair has yet to be determined.

References

[1] Buckwalter JA, Saltzman CL. Ankle osteoarthritis: distinctive characteristics. Instr Course Lect 1999;48:233–41.
[2] Saltzman CL, Salamon ML, Blanchard GM, et al. Report of a consecutive series of 639 patients from a tertiary orthopaedic center. Iowa Orthop J 2005;25:44–6.
[3] Coester LM, Saltzman CL, Leupold J, et al. Long-term results following ankle arthrodesis for post-traumatic arthritis. J Bone Joint Surg Am 2001;83:219–28.
[4] Giannini S, Buda R, Faldini C, et al. The treatment of severe posttraumatic arthritis of the ankle joint. J Bone Joint Surg Am 2007;89(Suppl 3):15–28.
[5] O'Driscoll SW, Saris DBF. Articular cartilage repair. In: Einhorn TA, O'Keefe RJ, Buckwalter JA, editors. Orthopaedic basic science: foundations of clinical practice. 3rd edition. Rosemont (IL): American Academy of Orthopedic Surgeons; 2007. p. 349–63.
[6] Schmidt MB, Chen EH, Lynch SE. A review of the effects of insulin-like growth factor and platelet derived growth factor on in vivo cartilage healing and repair. Osteoarthritis Cartilage 2006;14:403–12.
[7] Verschure PJ, van der Kraan PM, Vitters EL, et al. Stimulation of proteoglycan synthesis by triamcinolone acetonide and insulin-like growth factor 1 in normal and arthritic murine articular cartilage. J Rheumatol 1994;21:920–6.
[8] Jenniskens YM, Koevoet W, de Bart AC, et al. Biochemical and functional modulation of the cartilage collagen network by IGF1, TGFbeta2 and FGF2. Osteoarthritis Cartilage 2006;14:1136–46.
[9] Martin JA, Ellerbroek SM, Buckwalter JA. Age-related decline in chondrocyte response to insulin-like growth factor-I: the role of growth factor binding proteins. J Orthop Res 1997;15:491–8.
[10] Verschure PJ, Marle JV, Joosten LA, et al. Localization of insulin-like growth factor-1 receptor in human normal and osteoarthritic cartilage in relation to proteoglycan synthesis and content. Br J Rheumatol 1996;35:1044–55.
[11] Verschure PJ, Joosten LA, Van de Loo FA, et al. IL-1 has no direct role in the IGF-1 non-responsive state during experimentally induced arthritis in mouse knee joints. Ann Rheum Dis 1995;54:976–82.

[12] Verschure PJ, Joosten LA, van der Kraan PM, et al. Responsiveness of articular cartilage from normal and inflamed mouse knee joints to various growth factors. Ann Rheum Dis 1994;53:455–60.

[13] Verschure PJ, van Marle J, Joosten LA, et al. Localization and quantification of the insulin-like growth factor-1 receptor in mouse articular cartilage by confocal laser scanning microscopy. J Histochem Cytochem 1994;42:765–73.

[14] Verschure PJ, van Marle J, Joosten LA, et al. Chondrocyte IGF-1 receptor expression and responsiveness to IGF-1 stimulation in mouse articular cartilage during various phases of experimentally induced arthritis. Ann Rheum Dis 1995;54:645–53.

[15] Verschure PJ, Van Marle J, Joosten LA, et al. Histochemical analysis of insulin-like growth factor-1 binding sites in mouse normal and experimentally induced arthritic articular cartilage. Histochem J 1996;28:13–23.

[16] Nixon AJ, Lust G, Vernier-Singer M. Isolation, propagation, and cryopreservation of equine articular chondrocytes. Am J Vet Res 1992;53:2364–70.

[17] Nixon AJ, Fortier LA, Williams J, et al. Enhanced repair of extensive articular defects by insulin-like growth factor-I-laden fibrin composites. J Orthop Res 1999;17(4):475–87.

[18] Fortier LA, Mohammed HO, Lust G, et al. Insulin-like growth factor-I enhances cell-based repair of articular cartilage. J Bone Joint Surg Br 2002;84:276–88.

[19] Goodrich LR, Hidaka C, Robbins PD, et al. Genetic modification of chondrocytes with insulin-like growth factor-1 enhances cartilage healing in an equine model. J Bone Joint Surg Br 2007;89:672–85.

[20] Madry H, Kaul G, Cucchiarini M, et al. Enhanced repair of articular cartilage defects in vivo by transplanted chondrocytes overexpressing insulin-like growth factor I (IGF-I). Gene Ther 2005;12:1171–9.

[21] Morisset S, Frisbie DD, Robbins PD, et al. IL-1ra/IGF-1 gene therapy modulates repair of microfractured chondral defects. Clin Orthop Relat Res 2007;462:221–8.

[22] Rogachefsky RA, Dean DD, Howell DS, et al. Treatment of canine osteoarthritis with insulin-like growth factor-1 (IGF-1) and sodium pentosan polysulfate. Osteoarthritis Cartilage 1993;1:105–14.

[23] Reddi AH. Bone and cartilage differenciation. Curr Opin Genet Dev 1994;4(5):737–44.

[24] Urist MR. Bone: formation by autoinduction. Science 1965;150:893–9.

[25] Reddi AH, Huggins CB. Citrate and alkaline phosphatase during transformation of fibroblasts by the matrix and minerals of bone. Proc Soc Exp Biol Med 1972;140:807–10.

[26] Wozney JM, Rosen V. Bone morphogenic proteins and their gene expression. In: Noda M, editor. Cellular and Molecular Biology of Bone. San Diego (CA): Academy Press; 1993. p. 131–67.

[27] Mont MA, Ragland PS, Biggins B, et al. Use of bone morphogenetic proteins for musculoskeletal applications. An overview. J Bone Joint Surg Am 2004;86(Suppl 2):41–55.

[28] Chubinskaya S, Hurtig M, Rueger DC. OP-1/BMP-7 in cartilage repair. Int Orthop 2007;31(6):773–81.

[29] Fan Z, Chubinskaya S, Rueger D, et al. Regulation of anabolic and catabolic gene expression in normal and osteoarthritic adult human articular chondrocytes by osteogenic protein-1. Clin Exp Rheumatol 2004;22:103–6.

[30] Flechtenmacher J, Huch K, Thonar EJ, et al. Recombinant human osteogenic protein 1 is a potent stimulator of the synthesis of cartilage proteoglycans and collagens by human articular chondrocytes. Arthritis Rheum 1996;39:1896–904.

[31] Loeser RF, Pacione CA, Chubinskaya S. The combination of insulin-like growth factor 1 and osteogenic protein 1 promotes increased survival of and matrix synthesis by normal and osteoarthritic human articular chondrocytes. Arthritis Rheum 2003;48:2188–96.

[32] Nishida Y, Knudson CB, Eger W, et al. Osteogenic protein 1 stimulates cells-associated matrix assembly by normal human articular chondrocytes: up-regulation of hyaluronan synthase, CD44, and aggrecan. Arthritis Rheum 2000;43:206–14.

[33] Nishida Y, Knudson CB, Knudson W. Osteogenic protein-1 inhibits matrix depletion in a hyaluronan hexasaccharide-induced model of osteoarthritis. Osteoarthritis Cartilage 2004; 12(5):374–82.

[34] Chubinskaya S, Kumar B, Merrihew C, et al. Age-related changes in cartilage endogenous osteogenic protein-1 (OP-1). Biochim Biophys Acta 2002;1588:126–34.

[35] Merrihew C, Kumar B, Heretis K, et al. Alterations in endogenous osteogenic protein-1 with degeneration of human articular cartilage. J Orthop Res 2003;21:899–907.

[36] Grgic M, Jelic M, Basic V, et al. Regeneration of articular cartilage defects in rabbits by osteogenic protein-1 (bone morphogenetic protein-7). Acta Med Croatica 1997;51:23–7.

[37] Kuo AC, Rodrigo JJ, Reddi AH, et al. Microfracture and bone morphogenetic protein 7 (BMP-7) synergistically stimulate articular cartilage repair. Osteoarthritis Cartilage 2006; 14:1126–35.

[38] Mason JM, Breitbart AS, Barcia M, et al. Cartilage and bone regeneration using gene-enhanced tissue engineering. Clin Orthop Relat Res 2000;377(Suppl):S171–8.

[39] Cook SD, Patron LP, Salkeld SL, et al. Repair of articular cartilage defects with osteogenic protein-1 (BMP-7) in dogs. J Bone Joint Surg Am 2003;85(Suppl 3):116–23.

[40] Jelic M, Pecina M, Haspl M, et al. Regeneration of articular cartilage chondral defects by osteogenic protein-1 (bone morphogenetic protein-7) in sheep. Growth Factors 2001; 19(2):101–13.

[41] Hidaka C, Goodrich LR, Chen CT, et al. Acceleration of cartilage repair by genetically modified chondrocytes over expressing bone morphogenetic protein-7. J Orthop Res 2003;21(4): 573–83.

[42] Badlani N, Inoue A, Healey R, et al. The protective effect of OP-1 on articular cartilage in the development of osteoarthritis. Osteoarthritis Cartilage 2008;16(5):600–6.

[43] Hurtig MB, Chubinskaya S. The protective effect of OP-1 in early traumatic osteoarthritis-animal studies. Trans 5th ORS. 2004. p. 40.

[44] Im HJ, Pacione C, Chubinskaya S, et al. Inhibitory effects of insulin-like growth factor-1 and osteogenic protein-1 on fibronectin fragment- and interleukin-1{beta}-stimulated matrix metalloproteinase-13 expression in human chondrocytes. J Biol Chem 2003;278(28):25386–94.

[45] Hurtig MB. Delayed administration of OP-1 reduces articular degeneration after contusive impact injury. Transactions 5th ORS 2004;24:1338.

[46] Einhorn TA, Boskey AL, Gundeberg CM, et al. The mineral and mechanical properties of bone in chronic experimental diabetes. J Orthop Res 1988;6(3):317–23.

[47] Andrew JG, Hoyland JA, Freemont AJ, et al. Platelet-derived growth factor expression in normally healing human fractures. Bone 1995;16:455–60.

[48] Smith RJ, Justen JM, Sam LM, et al. Platelet-derived growth factor potentiates cellular responses of articular chondrocytes to interleukin-1. Arthritis Rheum 1991;34:697–706.

[49] Kieswetter K, Schwartz Z, Alderete M, et al. Platelet derived growth factor stimulates chondrocyte proliferation but prevents endochondral maturation. Endocrine 1997;6:257–64.

[50] Gaissmaier C, Fritz J, Krackhardt T, et al. Effect of human platelet supernatant on proliferation and matrix synthesis of human articular chondrocytes in monolayer and three-dimensional alginate cultures. Biomaterials 2005;26:1953–60.

[51] Lohmann CH, Schwartz Z, Niederauer GG, et al. Pretreatment with platelet derived growth factor-BB modulates the ability of costochondral resting zone chondrocytes incorporated into PLA/PGA scaffolds to form new cartilage in vivo. Biomaterials 2000;21:49–61.

[52] Fetter NL, Leddy HA, Guilak F, et al. Composition and transport properties of human ankle and knee cartilage. J Orthop Res 2006;24(2):211–9.

[53] Cole AA, Kuettner KE. Molecular basis for differences between human joints. Cell Mol Life Sci 2002;59(1):19–26.

[54] Aaron RK, Ciombor DM. Electrical stimulation of bone induction and grafting. In: Habal MB, editor. Bone grafts and bone substitutes. Philadelphia: WB Saunders; 1992. p. 192–205.

[55] Aaron RK, Ciombor DM, Simon BJ. Treatment of nonunions with electric and electromagnetic fields. Clin Orthop Relat Res 2004;(419):21–9.

[56] Fini M, Giavaresi G, Carpi A, et al. Effects of pulsed electromagnetic fields on articular hyaline cartilage: review of experimental and clinical studies. Biomed Pharmacother 2005;59: 388–94.

[57] Panagopoulos DJ, Karabarbounis A, Margaritis LH. Mechanism for action of electromagnetic fields on cells. Biochem Biophys Res Commun 2002;298:95–102.

[58] Luben RA, Cain CD, Chen MC, et al. Effects of electromagnetic stimuli on bone and bone cells in vitro: inhibition of responses to parathyroid hormone by low-energy low-frequency fields. Proc Natl Acad Sci U S A 1982;79:4180–4.

[59] Cain CD, Adey WR, Luben RA. Evidence that pulsed electromagnetic fields inhibit coupling of adenylate cyclase by parathyroid hormone in bone cells. J Bone Miner Res 1987;2:437–41.

[60] Hiraki Y, Endo N, Takigawa M, et al. Enhanced responsiveness to parathyroid hormone and induction of functional differentiation of cultured rabbit costal chondrocytes by a pulsed electromagnetic field. Biochim Biophys Acta 1987;931:94–100.

[61] Aaron RK, Boyan BD, Ciombor DM, et al. Stimulation of growth factor synthesis by electric and electromagnetic fields. Clin Orthop Relat Res 2004;(419):30–7.

[62] Fanelli C, Coppola S, Barone R, et al. Magnetic fields increase cell survival by inhibiting apoptosis via modulation of Ca2+ influx. FASEB J 1999;13:95–102.

[63] Lorich DG, Brighton CT, Gupta R, et al. Biochemical pathway mediating the response of bone cells to capacitive coupling. Clin Orthop Relat Res 1998;(350):246–56.

[64] Nagai M, Ota M. Pulsating electromagnetic field stimulates mRNA expression of bone morphogenetic protein-2 and -4. J Dent Res 1994;73:1601–5.

[65] Zhuang H, Wang W, Seldes RM, et al. Electrical stimulation induces the level of TGF-beta1 mRNA in osteoblastic cells by a mechanism involving calcium/calmodulin pathway. Biochem Biophys Res Commun 1997;237:225–9.

[66] Aaron RK, Wang S, Ciombor DM. Upregulation of basal TGF-beta1 levels by EMF coincident with chondrogenesis–implications for skeletal repair and tissue engineering. J Orthop Res 2002;20:233–40.

[67] Sakai A, Suzuki K, Nakamura T, et al. Effects of pulsing electromagnetic fields on cultured cartilage cells. Int Orthop 1991;15:341–6.

[68] De Mattei M, Caruso A, Pezzetti F, et al. Effects of pulsed electromagnetic fields on human articular chondrocyte proliferation. Connect Tissue Res 2001;42:269–79.

[69] Fioravanti A, Nerucci F, Collodel G, et al. Biochemical and morphological study of human articular chondrocytes cultivated in the presence of pulsed signal therapy. Ann Rheum Dis 2002;61:1032–3.

[70] Ciombor DM, Aaron RK, Wang S, et al. Modification of osteoarthritis by pulsed electromagnetic field–a morphological study. Osteoarthritis Cartilage 2003;11:455–62.

[71] van Beuningen HM, van der Kraan PM, Arntz OJ, et al. Protection from interleukin 1 induced destruction of articular cartilage by transforming growth factor beta: studies in anatomically intact cartilage in vitro and in vivo. Ann Rheum Dis 1993;52:185–91.

[72] van Beuningen HM, van der Kraan PM, Arntz OJ, et al. Transforming growth factor-beta 1 stimulates articular chondrocyte proteoglycan synthesis and induces osteophyte formation in the murine knee joint. Lab Invest 1994;71:279–90.

[73] Fini M, Giavaresi G, Torricelli P, et al. Pulsed electromagnetic fields reduce knee osteoarthritic lesion progression in the aged Dunkin Hartley guinea pig. J Orthop Res 2005;23: 899–908.

[74] Fini M, Torricelli P, Giavaresi G, et al. Effect of pulsed electromagnetic field stimulation on knee cartilage, subchondral and epyphiseal trabecular bone of aged Dunkin Hartley guinea pigs. Biomed Pharmacother 2007;10.1016/j.biopha.2007.03.001.

[75] Zizic TM, Hoffman KC, Holt PA, et al. The treatment of osteoarthritis of the knee with pulsed electrical stimulation. J Rheumatol 1995;22:1757–61.

[76] Trock DH, Bollet AJ, Markoll R. The effect of pulsed electromagnetic fields in the treatment of osteoarthritis of the knee and cervical spine. Report of randomized, double blind, placebo controlled trials. J Rheumatol 1994;21:1903–11.

[77] Pipitone N, Scott DL. Magnetic pulse treatment for knee osteoarthritis: a randomised, double-blind, placebo-controlled study. Curr Med Res Opin 2001;17:190–6.
[78] Hulme J, Robinson V, DeBie R, et al. Electromagnetic fields for the treatment of osteoarthritis. Cochrane Database Syst Rev 2002;CD003523.

ELSEVIER
SAUNDERS

Foot Ankle Clin N Am
13 (2008) 381–400

FOOT AND
ANKLE CLINICS

Ankle Arthrodesis: The Simple and the Complex

Jamal Ahmad, MD*, Steven M. Raikin, MD

*Rothman Institute Orthopaedics at Thomas Jefferson University Hospital,
925 Chestnut Street, Philadelphia, PA 19107, USA*

The ankle joint is a constrained mortise-and-tenon type joint consisting of the distal tibial plafond and fibula articulating with the dome of the talus. Arthritis of the ankle can result in pain, joint incongruence, decreased motion, and functional disability. Most ankle arthritis is posttraumatic, a category that includes cartilaginous injury and ligamentous insufficiency [1]. Other less common causes of arthritis include talar osteonecrosis, infection, and Charcot neuroarthropathy [2].

The current standard surgical treatment for arthritis that has not responded to nonoperative management is joint arthrodesis. Ankle arthrodesis was described first by Albert [3] in 1879. Since then, the procedure has received numerous modifications to address different types of clinical situations with different levels of complexity. Scenarios that involve minimal challenges are patients who have posttraumatic arthritis, mild-to-moderate deformity, and minimal bone loss. These patients are amenable to a transfibular open ankle arthrodesis with some type of internal fixation. For patients who have no or minimal deformity, arthroscopic and minimally invasive "mini-open" ankle arthrodeses with percutaneous screws also are treatment options.

Other clinical scenarios present greater challenges in achieving a successful ankle arthrodesis. As deformity from posttraumatic arthritis worsens, patients can develop significant bone loss and adjacent hindfoot joint (ie, subtalar and talonavicular) arthritis that also requires treatment. Talar osteonecrosis and Charcot neuroarthropathy are special circumstances that can lead to bone loss and arthritis distal to the ankle. Postinfectious ankle arthritis can present with varying amounts of deformity and bone loss.

---

* Corresponding author.
  E-mail address: jamal.ahmad@rothmaninstitute.com (J. Ahmad).

1083-7515/08/$ - see front matter © 2008 Elsevier Inc. All rights reserved.
doi:10.1016/j.fcl.2008.04.007   *foot.theclinics.com*

This situation is complex, because the surgeon must achieve a solid fusion and also eliminate infection.

In addition, the indications for ankle arthrodesis have broadened from solely addressing arthritis. In certain instances a fusion can be used as a leg-salvage procedure to avoid a below-knee amputation (BKA). Such indications include failure of total ankle arthroplasty (TAA), surgical management following periarticular tumor resection, and talar extrusion following high-energy trauma (Box 1).

Preoperative planning

Preoperative planning begins with a thorough assessment of the patient's medical and social history, especially medication and tobacco use, and an assessment of potential infection in the ankle joint. If a joint infection is suspected, preoperative laboratory values are critical and include an erythrocyte sedimentation rate, C-reactive protein level, and full blood cell counts.

Weight-bearing radiographs of the ankle in the anteroposterior, lateral, and mortise plane are important in planning an ankle arthrodesis. Weight-bearing films allow more accurate evaluation of malalignment and loss of joint space [4]. It also is important to assess the foot for other areas of arthritis, particularly the subtalar, Chopart, and midfoot joints, because involvement of these articulations may alter the choice of procedure and method. If the foot is involved, weight-bearing radiographs of the foot in the anteroposterior, lateral, and oblique plane should be performed as well.

The alignment of the whole leg needs to be assessed, because it may affect the final positioning of the proposed arthrodesis procedure. If there is

---

Box 1. Indications and contraindications for isolated ankle arthrodesis

Indications for isolated ankle joint arthrodesis
Advanced arthritic involvement of the ankle joint
Unstable Charcot neuroarthropathic ankle joint

Contraindications for isolated ankle joint arthrodesis
Absolute contraindications
    Vascular status of region inadequate for bone/incision healing
Relative contraindications
    Bilateral ankle arthritis (difficulty rising out of chair/climbing
        stairs/walking on inclines)
    Involvement of subtalar/Chopart joints (requires
        tibiotalocalcaneal or pantalar arthrodesis)
    Significant osteonecrosis of talus or distal tibia
    Open physeal plates (will result in premature growth arrest)

a history of prior limb trauma, long-plate whole-limb radiographs may be required. At the very least, the tibial alignment should be visualized (and corrected if abnormal) in all cases.

Open transfibular ankle arthrodesis

Currently, the most common surgical exposure for open ankle arthrodesis is the lateral transfibular approach. Upon osteotomy, the distal fibula can be used either as bone graft or as a lateral strut to increase the stability of the arthrodesis construct. Preparations of the distal tibia and talar dome are performed as either "dome" cuts or flat cuts. Dome cuts allow minimal loss of height but offer little opportunity for angular correction. Straight, flat cuts allow correction of significant deformity but can result in loss of joint height. Care is taken to preserve the medial malleolus unless its presence interferes with deformity correction.

The ankle should be fused in 5° of valgus, 0° of dorsiflexion, and 10° of external rotation [5]. This position is best, because it results in a plantigrade foot and maximal functional results [6]. Once this alignment is obtained, the ankle arthrodesis commonly is held with three 6.5- or 7.3-mm short-threaded, cannulated, cancellous screws [7,8]. An ankle arthrodesis achieved with three screws has greater biomechanical rigidity than one using two screws [9–11]. A method of using three screws involves two crossing screws and a third posterior-to-anterior (PA) "home run" screw [1,12]. Laboratory tests have shown that a crossing configuration of the first two screws is stiffer than parallel screw placement (Fig. 1) [12,13].

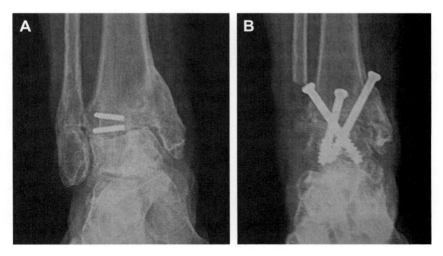

Fig. 1. (A) Preoperative and (B) postoperative radiographs of a patient who received an open transfibular ankle arthrodesis. Note the preoperative varus alignment and mild bone loss in panel A. The distal fibula is morselized and used as bone graft.

There are many reports of long-term follow-up of this technique of ankle arthrodesis as it is commonly used. Fusion rates range from 75% to 100% by 12 weeks postoperatively [14–16]. Relief of symptoms is highly predictable, and patient satisfaction rates as high as 90% are reported [15,17].

Aside from large-diameter screws, alternative other fixation devices to achieve arthrodesis include large-fragment T-plates, staples, Ilizarov external fixation, screws combined with cables in a tension-band construct, and tibiotalar intramedullary nails [18–22]. Some other constructs, including blade plates and anteriorly placed large-fragment plates, have been tested to date only in biomechanical studies [13,23].

Arthroscopic ankle arthrodesis

When there is minimal or no deformity or bone loss, arthroscopic ankle arthrodesis is an alternative technique [24–26]. The advantages of this newer procedure are (1) decreased incision size to minimize morbidity, which includes the risks of skin slough, wound dehiscence, and postoperative infection; (2) distal fibula preservation; and (3) preservation of the peroneal artery, which may affect healing of the fusion positively.

For this procedure, a standard two- or three-portal ankle arthroscopy is performed. With the joint distracted, the articular cartilage and subchondral bone is removed with curettes and mechanical burrs. Two or three percutaneous cannulated cancellous screws then are placed across the ankle under fluoroscopic guidance to achieve fusion.

Since the procedure first was described in 1983, several authors have reported their experience. Ogilvie-Harris and colleagues [27] presented an 89% union rate among 19 arthroscopic fusions with a mean time to union of 10.5 weeks. Zvijac and colleagues [28] reported a 95% union rate among 21 arthroscopic fusions with an average time to fusion of 8.9 weeks. Myerson and Quill [29] retrospectively compared arthroscopic versus open arthrodesis in 33 patients. The arthroscopic group showed 100% union at a mean of 8.7 weeks; the open population displayed a 94% union rate at a mean of 14.5 weeks after surgery. Patients who had more deformity or osteonecrosis were placed selectively in the open population, however, because of the study's inherent retrospective nature. In one of the largest studies to date, Winson and colleagues [30] described a non-union rate of 7.6% in 105 arthroscopic ankle arthrodeses.

The technique of arthroscopic ankle arthrodesis has shortcomings, however. The technique itself is technically demanding and has a steep learning curve [1]. Because a burr is used to prepare the distal tibia and talar dome surfaces, there is a genuine concern about thermal injury to the bony surfaces, which can increase the risk of non-union [31].

Minimally invasive ankle arthrodesis

To combine the advantages of the open and arthroscopic ankle fusion methods while limiting their respective disadvantages, a minimally invasive or "mini-open" technique has been proposed as an alternative for patients who have minimal or no deformity or bone loss. The advantages of this newer procedure are (1) decreased incision sizes to minimize morbidity, which include the risks of skin slough, wound dehiscence, and postoperative infection; (2) distal fibula preservation; (3) preservation of the peroneal artery; (4) elimination of burrs to prepare bony surfaces, which otherwise could cause thermal necrosis; and (5) decreased time to union.

Two 2-cm vertical incisions centered over the standard portal sites for ankle arthroscopy are used for this technique. The anteromedial incision is made immediately medial to the tibialis anterior tendon, between the tendon and the notch of the medial malleolus. The anterolateral incision is made in the space between the lateral border of the peroneus tertius tendon and the anterior border of the fibula. The articular cartilage and subchondral bone is removed through these incisions with curettes and chisels. Neither power saws nor burrs are used to limit potential thermal necrosis of the bone that may lead to non-union of the arthrodesis. Two or three percutaneous, cannulated, cancellous screws then are placed across the ankle under fluoroscopic guidance to achieve fusion (Fig. 2A, B).

To date, limited published data exist for the mini-open ankle arthrodesis. Myerson and colleagues [31,32] described the procedure and published their results in two separate studies. Miller and colleagues [32] performed this type of fusion on 32 ankles and describe a 96.8% union rate with an average time to union of 8 weeks. Paremain and colleagues [31] separately reported a union rate of 100% at a mean time of 6 weeks (range, 3–15 weeks) in 15 ankles.

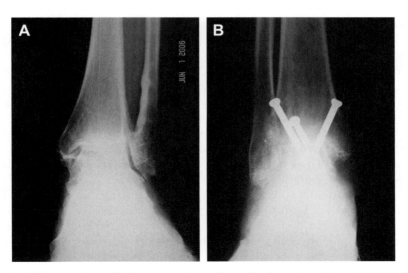

Fig. 2. (A) Preoperative and (B) postoperative radiographs of a patient who received a "mini-open" ankle arthrodesis. The normal alignment and the absence of the bone loss seen in Fig. 1A make this type of procedure appropriate for this patient.

Alternative surgical approaches

Many patients who have posttraumatic ankle arthritis have undergone prior and often multiple surgical procedures. These patients can have such involved incisions that a standard lateral approach to the ankle is precluded, because it could generate wound-healing problems requiring plastic surgical coverage. In such situations, alternate approaches such as a posterior approach described by Gruen and Mears [33] or a direct anterior approach may be used better. An additional advantage of the anterior approach is that the fibula can be spared to allow potential conversion to an arthroplasty in the future. Furthermore, most arthroplasties currently are performed through an anterior approach, allowing conversion to be performed through this same incision in the future.

Complex situations

Increasing deformity with adjacent joint arthritis

When evaluating patients who have ankle arthritis and complex deformity, it also is important to assess the hindfoot for degenerative change. As ankle arthritis and deformity worsen, increased forces are transmitted through the subtalar and talonavicular joints and result in degenerative changes. In turn, patients initially may develop a rigid planovalgus foot deformity and only hindfoot arthritis caused by conditions such as posterior tibial tendon dysfunction [34,35]. With worsening valgus deformity at the hindfoot, the deltoid ligament becomes incompetent, often causing rigid ankle deformity and arthritis [36,37]. With arthritis and deformity at both the ankle and hindfoot, one must appreciate the increased complexity, because the methods of achieving an ankle arthrodesis must be altered to treat the hindfoot [38].

When patients develop disease at the ankle and subtalar joints, the current standard treatment is a tibiotalocalcaneal (TTC) arthrodesis. Both lateral transfibular and posterior approaches to expose the ankle and subtalar joints have been described. The posterior has the theoretic advantage over the lateral transfibular approach of less potential injury to the talar blood supply and increased visualization and possible correction of coronal plane deformities [39]. These advantages have yet to be proven in clinical studies.

A variety of materials have been used to obtain a TTC arthrodesis [40–42]. Russotti and colleagues [43] used multiple screws or an external fixator to achieve a TTC fusion. They reported satisfactory results in 16 of 21 patients (76%) and bony union in 18 of 21 patients (86%). Other authors have turned to more rigid retrograde intramedullary nails for TTC arthrodeses. Kile and colleagues [44] presented satisfactory results in 26 of 30 patients (87%) and bony union in 28 of 30 patients (93%) who received an intramedullary nail for the fusion. Chou and colleagues [45] conducted a multicenter retrospective study involving 37 patients who received an intramedullary nail for a TTC arthrodesis, 32 of whom (86.5%) progressed to bony union. Mendicino and colleagues [40] performed 20 TTC arthrodeses with an intramedullary nail and reported bony union in 19 of the 20 fusions (95%). In the same study, however, they report 5 patients (25%) had major complications, and 11 (55%) had minor postoperative complications. Because more TTC arthrodeses were being done with an intramedullary nail, Chiodo and colleagues [46] compared the use of an intramedullary nail with blade plate-and-screw fixation for TTC fusion in an osteopenic cadaveric model. They found the blade plate-and-screw model had a significantly higher mean initial and final stiffness and decreased plastic deformation. Hanson and Cracchiolo [47] performed 10 TTC arthrodeses using a posterior approach and a blade plate. They report successful results, with all patients achieving a solid fusion by a mean time of 14.5 weeks and excellent pain relief. Blade plates, however, can be technically challenging with little room for error, and their screws do not offer multiple planes of fixation [48]. Locking plates are easier to use than blade plates. Through their unique design, they act as a fixed-angle device with the locking screws providing fixation in multiple planes. There is only one study regarding the clinical use of a locking plate for a TTC fusion. Ahmad and colleagues [49] used a proximal humerus locking plate to perform 18 TTC arthrodeses in 17 patients. They report a union rate of 94.4% by a mean time of 20.7 weeks in complex and revision cases.

Although a TTC fusion is appropriate for treating complex disease and deformity at both the ankle and subtalar joints, there currently is no standard implant for this procedure. Each implant is best for specific scenarios, depending on inherent complexity. Screws are best reserved for situations with minimal deformity. Although they are simple to use, they may not provide enough compression and stability when there is significant deformity [50]. Thin-wire external fixation may confer sufficient stability as long as it is truly multiplanar. These devices are at risk for pin tract infection, however. Patients who have severe bone loss from deformity may be suited better for an intramedullary nail. Blade plates and locking plates are highly rigid devices that can be advantageous in osteopenic patients. Locking plates have added benefits, because they act as a fixed-angle device with the locking screws acting as multiplanar fixation.

When patients have talonavicular joint arthritis and deformity with ankle and subtalar disease, the orthopaedic treatment must be a pantalar arthrodesis. The ankle and subtalar joints still are addressed as a TTC fusion. Then the talonavicular joint usually is fused with two 4.0- or 4.5-mm cannulated screws through a longitudinal medial surgical approach [51]. In more complex circumstances in which the joint is osteopenic, compression staples may be used with or in place of screws across the joint. Papa and Myerson [52] performed eight pantalar fusions with compression screws and report a 62.5% union rate. More recently, Acosta and colleagues [48] performed 14 pantalar fusions and report a higher union rate of 71.4%. Although both groups report that most of their respective patients were satisfied with the final outcome of the procedure, they acknowledge the complexity of treating such difficult cases of arthritis and deformity.

Talar osteonecrosis

The primary causes of talar osteonecrosis are trauma, medications, and vaso-occlusive diseases. The types of injuries that most often progress to osteonecrosis are talar neck and body fractures or peritalar dislocations. Because of its unique but well described extraosseous and intraosseous blood supply and anatomy, the talus is susceptible to posttraumatic osteonecrosis [53–55]. The two most common medications linked to talar osteonecrosis are steroids and chemotherapeutic drugs. Vaso-occlusive disease states that can cause osteonecrosis include hyperlipidemia, sickle cell disease, and lupus.

Both radiographs and MRI of the ankle should be used to evaluate the talus for osteonecrosis. Early radiographic signs of osteonecrosis include an increase in talar body bone density and relative osteoporosis of surrounding necrotic bone. As the osteonecrosis worsens, talar collapse and degenerative changes at the peritalar joints ensue. On MRI, osteonecrosis appears as patchy or serpentine edema. MRI is most useful in quantifying the amount of osteonecrosis.

Several investigators have recently modified the Ficat and Arlet classification for femoral head osteonecrosis to classify the disease at the talus [56]:

Stage I: positive changes only on technetium bone scan or MRI
Stage II: subchondral sclerosis without talar collapse
Stage III: bony collapse of the talus without degenerative changes at tibiotalar or subtalar joints
Stage IV: talar collapse and degenerative changes at the tibiotalar and/or subtalar joints

Current treatment of talar osteonecrosis depends on its stage and the distribution of the osteonecrosis within the talar dome, which may be patchy. Management of stage I or II osteonecrosis is directed toward preventing talar collapse and avoiding ankle arthrodesis. This management includes nonsurgical means such as limiting weight bearing in a patellar tendon–bearing brace and newer operative methods, such as core decompression and bone grafting [57–60], which are beyond the scope of this article. When osteonecrosis has progressed to stage III or IV with talar collapse, ankle arthrodesis may become necessary. Surgical steps that are critical to obtaining a successful arthrodesis include removal of entire portions of the talus that are necrotic, ensuring enough compression and stability of fixation across the ankle joint, and the use of bone autograft or allograft as a bioadjuvant.

If only the tibiotalar joint is involved, and enough vascularity persists within the talar body and neck, tibiotalar fusion with bone grafting can be performed. If enough viable bone remains within the talar body, screws alone can be used to achieve compression across the ankle joint. When there is greater bone loss because of osteonecrosis, plates, intramedullary devices, or external fixators are better at ensuring ankle stability and rigidity.

If most of the talar body is osteonecrotic and needs to be excised, an alternative means of fusing the tibiotalar joint is a modified Blair fusion. In 1943, Blair [61] described a method of primarily fusing the ankle joint to treat comminuted talar fractures that involves removal of talar body and sliding the anterior distal tibial cortex distally to create an onlay graft into the talar neck. Several authors have modified this technique with internal fixation to fuse the ankle joint and to treat osteonecrosis simultaneously, but results have been mixed. Morris [62] performed the modified Blair fusion in four patients and reported a 100% union rate with minimal pain at final follow-up. Two separate studies were unable to repeat these results. Dennis and Tullos [63] report a non-union rate of 29% in seven patients. Van Bergeyk and colleagues [64] describe the same non-union rate with some patients having persistent pain in long-term follow-up. Several authorities express reservations about this procedure [65]. When the talar body is to be removed for this procedure, the posterior articular facet of the subtalar joint is sacrificed, thereby increasing the contact forces of the anterior and middle facets and increasing the risk of future degenerative subtalar arthritis. Although the modified Blair fusion may be appropriate for some patients, in many instances the degree of osteonecrosis and bone loss is too great to treat in this manner.

In these more advanced cases, the preferred surgery is a TTC arthrodesis with bone grafting [66]. This procedure can include using a bulk allograft such as a femoral head or a tricortical iliac crest autograft to replace the missing portion of the talar body and prevent excessive limb shortening. As previously mentioned, several devices can be used for a TTC arthrodesis. Although there is no standard implant, retrograde intramedullary nails currently may be best suited for patients who have severe osteonecrosis. Nail fixation can overcome severe bone loss through proximal and distal locking of the nail. Talar body reaming during nail insertion may have a theoretic advantage of talar decompression and potential revascularization. The literature to date does not conclusively favor one type of implant over another for TTC fusion in this context, however.

In fact, there is scant research regarding the use of a TTC arthrodesis to treat talar osteonecrosis. Kitaoka and colleagues [65] performed 14 TTC fusions in 14 patients: external fixation in 10 patients, compression staples in 3 patients, and no fixation in the last patient. They report a union rate of 78.6%, with two non-unions in the external fixation group and the third non-union in the patient who had no fixation. More recently, Ahmad and colleagues [49] used a locking plate for a TTC fusion in two patients who had talar osteonecrosis that progressed to complete union. Clearly, the specific role of a TTC arthrodesis in the management of osteonecrosis requires further investigation (Fig. 3A–E).

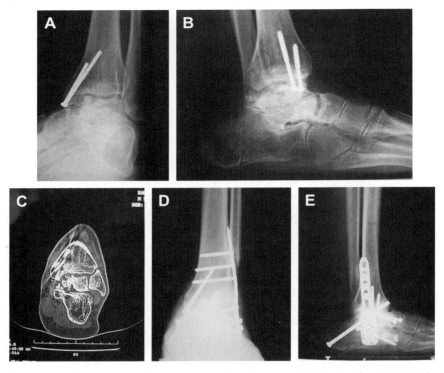

Fig. 3. (*A, B*) Preoperative radiographs of a patient who has posttraumatic talar osteonecrosis. (*C*) Preoperative CT scan of the same patient which shows the osteonecrosis to involve the entire medial half of the talar body. (*D, E*) Postoperative radiographs of the same patient after having received a pantalar fusion with a locking plate.

An alternate arthrodesis that has been described for treatment of talar osteonecrosis with nearly complete or complete bone loss is a talectomy with a tibiocalcaneal (TC) fusion [67]. Mann and Chou [68] performed this procedure in one patient using large-diameter screws. They state this patient developed a solid fusion by 3 months after surgery. Myerson and colleagues [69] also performed a talectomy and TC fusion in one patient but used an adolescent condylar blade plate. They also report a successful result, because this patient progressed to union. More recently, and with a larger patient population, Dennison and colleagues [70] performed six talectomies with TC fusions in six patients via Ilizarov external fixation and report a 100% union rate. This procedure has shortcomings, however. The primary fault of a TC fusion is a discrepancy in postoperative leg length. Dennison and colleagues overcame this problem by performing a concomitant distal tibial corticotomy and bone transport through the Ilizarov fixator. In addition, TC fixation is dependent on bone quality, which may be poor in patients who have significant osteopenia or osteoporosis.

Postinfectious arthritis

Infection is a rare but serious cause of ankle arthritis. Ankle joint infection most commonly occurs as the result of prior surgery, open wounds such as ulcers, and penetrating trauma such as degloving injuries and open fractures. Once the joint becomes infected, the cartilage is at high risk for bacterial enzymatic degradation. As infection worsens and joint cartilage is destroyed, the infection can spread to the distal tibial and/or talar bone. The treatment of such infection is complex, because the surgeon must not only address ankle arthritis and also must eradicate infection and manage bone loss in cases of osteomyelitis (Fig. 4).

In patients who had remote prior infections, standard fusion with internal fixation can be performed. A biopsy sent for frozen section histology can be performed intra-operatively, and if residual infection is present, the procedure can be staged with an initial irrigation and debridement with antibiotic spacer followed by later fusion or altered to a fusion using compression external fixation. In recent or currently active periarticular infection, the current preferred treatment involves complete debridement of infected material followed by ankle arthrodesis with an external fixator [71]. This treatment can be performed as a single or two-stage procedure. Kollig and colleagues [72] performed 15 ankle fusions in this manner and report a union rate of 93%. More recently, Saltzman [73] fused eight ankles with a union rate of 87.5%. Both authors remark that many of their patients had concurrent medical comorbidities and systemic illness, which can complicate the

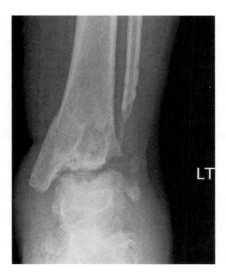

Fig. 4. A patient who has postinfectious ankle arthritis. Note the significant bone loss at the distal fibula, cavitary changes within the distal tibia, and sclerosis within the talar dome that increase the complexity of performing an ankle arthrodesis.

ankle arthrodesis and its healing. Although much of the literature to date is limited to case series, external fixators are best for these complex situations of postinfectious arthritis, because internal hardware may be at risk for infection.

An alternate arthrodesis that has been described for treatment of postinfectious arthritis with complete talar osteomyelitis is a talectomy with a TC fusion. Kolker and Wilson [74] performed a TC fusion in four patients who had external fixation and autogenous bone graft. They report a 100% union rate by 14 weeks and uniform good results. Little else has been published regarding this type of ankle arthrodesis in this setting, however.

Complete removal of infected material may require multiple debridements. If there are soft tissue defects after debridement, ankle arthrodesis is even more challenging. Depending on their size and depth, soft tissue deficiencies can be addressed with flap coverage (free or rotational) and skin grafting [75]. Within this complex setting, consultation with an experienced plastic surgeon can be invaluable.

Charcot neuroarthropathy

Charcot neuroarthropathy at the ankle is characterized by simultaneous fracture, bony collapse, and ultimately joint destruction. This condition occurs primarily in neuropathic patients who have some history of trauma. Currently, the most common cause of Charcot ankle neuroarthropathy is diabetes, and such patients often have low bone densities resulting from diabetic sequelae such as vascular disease and nephropathy. Charcot ankle neuroarthropathy can be difficult for the surgeon to manage. In addition to the deformity, instability, and bone loss, the surgeon must confront the patients' medical comorbidities, which can affect the success of an ankle arthrodesis deleteriously (Fig. 5).

The current standard treatment for a Charcot ankle that has not responded nonoperative management is ankle arthrodesis. The type and method of fusion can vary, however, depending on adjacent joint involvement and presence of infection. When patients present with isolated tibiotalar joint involvement and minimal bone loss, the preferred surgery is a transfibular ankle fusion with cross screw or plate fixation. Blade plates and, more recently, locking plates have been used in this scenario. The advantages of these implants over conventional plates have been described earlier: they are highly rigid in osteopenic patients. It is important to note the direction of patients' ankle instability, because dual plating may be necessary to confer sufficient ankle stability.

Management of Charcot ankle neuroarthropathy becomes even more complex, because the disease presents with adjacent joint arthritis, increased deformity, and progressive bone loss. When both the tibiotalar and subtalar joints are affected, the preferred surgery is a TTC arthrodesis with bone grafting. Various types of implants have been used for this purpose. Ahmad

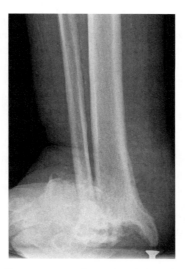

Fig. 5. A patient who has Charcot neuroarthropathy of the ankle. Note the significant bone loss at the talus that causes this ankle to be highly unstable. This is a complex situation to manage when performing an ankle arthrodesis.

and colleagues [49] used a locking plate in six patients and report a union rate of 83.3%. Some authors have used an intramedullary nail for a TTC fusion with reported union rates ranging from 71% to 78% [76,77]. Others have used external fixators as their primary choice of fixation, but publications remain limited to anecdotal experience [20,78–80]. Aside from these reports, there is little in the literature to date regarding the long-term results of TTC fusions for treatment of Charcot ankle arthropathy.

An alternate arthrodesis that has been described for treatment of Charcot ankle neuroarthropathy with nearly complete or complete talar bone loss is a talectomy with a TC arthrodesis. This procedure also has been performed using various kinds of implants. Myerson and colleagues [69] used a blade plate to perform 26 TC fusions and report a union rate of 92.3%. Pinzur and Noonan [81] performed TC arthrodeses in nine patients, all of whom progressed to complete union. Fabrin and colleagues [80] used external fixation in five patients but were unable to reproduce these results; their reported union rate was 20%. Aside from these case series, little has been reported regarding the role of TC arthrodesis in treating complex Charcot disease.

As ankle deformity worsens because of neuroarthropathy, patients may develop ulceration that ultimately can lead to soft tissue infection and osteomyelitis. Under such circumstances, the ankle arthrodesis is performed after debridement of infected material and with external fixation, as described in the previous section. Although Charcot disease itself is challenging to treat, the treatment becomes more complex in the presence of active infection.

Augmentation of the arthrodesis in the presence of Charcot neuroarthropathy usually is recommended. Many of these patients have poor-quality bone, and autograft bone may be of inadequate quality to ensure fusion. Using implantable electromagnetic bone stimulators at the time of surgery can increase the fusion rate in such complex patients [82].

Salvage after failure of total ankle arthroplasty

During the past several years, TAA has been performed increasingly to manage ankle arthritis. With the newer generation of arthroplasty, the documented 10-year survival rate for TAA ranges between 63% and 91% [83]. It is important to understand that TAA can have different complications than seen with ankle arthrodesis. Like most joint arthroplasties, the main complications seen following TAA include periprosthetic infection, instability, and subsidence [84–86]. TAA failure for any cause clearly is a complex situation to manage if the surgeon must confront joint infection and/or bone loss.

When the TAA fails because of infection, the arthrodesis is done in a staged manner [87]. The first step of treatment involves removal of prosthetic components and infected material, joint and soft tissue debridement, and temporary ankle stabilization. Often, complete removal of infected material may require multiple debridements. Soft tissue deficits at the ankle after debridement can be addressed with flap coverage (free or rotational) and skin grafting. Consultation with an experienced plastic surgeon can be invaluable in this complex setting. The ankle joint itself is stabilized temporarily with thin-wire external fixation and an antibiotic-impregnated polymethyl-methacrylate cement spacer to minimize dead space. After complete eradication of infection, the joint is fused. The best-described technique for arthrodesis in this scenario is continued use of external fixation with adjuvant bone grafting to manage bone loss [88]. One of the largest case series to date is that of Carlsson and colleagues [89] in which four patients who had infected TAAs were converted to an arthrodesis in this staged manner. They report a union rate of 100% with the remaining living patients being satisfied with the final outcome.

When the TAA fails from noninfectious causes, conversion to an ankle arthrodesis can be done in a single-stage procedure. If there are minimal bone defects following component removal, the authors propose isolated ankle joint fusion with bone grafting. Gabrion and colleagues [90] converted six failed TAAs to an ankle arthrodesis with an anterior plate and report successful results. Hopgood and colleagues [91] performed isolated ankle fusions in eight patients who had failed TAAs and minimal bone loss. They report a union rate of 100% in this population using compression screw fixation and bone grafting. Most recently, Culpan and colleagues [92] converted 16 failed TAAs to an ankle arthrodesis using internal fixation and bone graft. They report a union rate of 93.8%, noting that the one nonunion occurred in a patient who had significant bone loss.

When there is significant bone loss following TAA removal, a TTC fusion with bone grafting is recommended as treatment. Johl and colleagues [93] converted a failed TAA to a TTC fusion with an intramedullary nail and bone graft. They report that the patient progressed to union without complications. When faced with more extensive bone loss in their population of 23 patients who had failed TAAs, Hopgood and colleagues [91] performed 15 TTC arthrodeses; the remaining 8 patients, who had only minimal bone loss, received ankle fusions. The first 5 of these 15 patients received compression screws for a TTC fusion, but only 1 of these 5 (20%) progressed to union. Because of this poor success rate, the authors used an intramedullary nail to achieve a TTC arthrodesis in the remaining 10 patients and report a union rate of 80% (8 of 10). They conclude that although management of TAA failure with significant bone loss is challenging, the use of an intramedullary nail is the best means of achieving arthrodesis. More recently, Schill [94] converted 15 failed TAAs to TTC fusions with an intramedullary nail and bone autograft. They report a union rate of 93.3% with a wide range of patient satisfaction [91].

Certainly, ankle arthrodesis can be attempted to salvage the leg and avoid a BKA in this situation. No long-term studies assessing functional outcomes and ultimate satisfaction in patients undergoing conversion to TTC as compared with BKA for failed TAA are available, however. This situation may change as more TAAs are performed.

Limb salvage after tumor resection

Recently, some authors have described performing an ankle arthrodesis as a way to salvage the leg following surgical resection of distal tibial tumors. Using an ankle fusion in this manner is complex, because surgeons must address significant bone loss following tumor excision. Castro and colleagues [95] present a case report in which a patient who had a distal tibial osteosarcoma was treated with a TTC fusion with an intramedullary nail following a wide resection of the tumor. The patient had no tumor recurrence and progressed to complete union of the TTC fusion. Moore and colleagues [96] present a larger case series in which nine patients who had malignant distal tibial tumors were treated with a TTC fusion and bone allograft after a wide excision. They used an intramedullary nail to perform the fusion and report tumor recurrence in only one patient. Although this method of ankle arthrodesis as a means of limb salvage does offer an alternative over a BKA, its use certainly requires further long-term study.

Talar extrusion

Complete extrusion of the talus is a severe and rare injury. These situations become particularly difficult to manage when the talus is unavailable for reimplantation, because the surgeon must address both instability and bone loss at the ankle. To date, treatment of this complex injury remains limited to case reports. These same authors describe performing a delayed or immediate TC arthrodesis as a way to salvage the leg following these injuries. Hiraizumi and colleagues [97] performed a delayed TC fusion to treat pain and instability in a patient who previously had received a talectomy as immediate treatment for an extruded talus. They report that after union of the TC fusion this patient's symptoms improved substantially. More recently, Koller and colleagues [98] presented a case report in which two patients received a TC fusion with bone grafting as immediate treatment. They reported favorable outcomes, because both patients had minimal pain and progressed to complete union. Although the definitive treatment of total talar extrusion remains controversial because of its rarity, TC fusions seem to provide predictable pain relief and stability.

Summary

Patient factors determine whether an ankle arthrodesis is simple or complex. In cases of minimal or moderate ankle deformity with minimal bone loss, use of a transfibular ankle arthrodesis has proven to be reliable and reproducible in obtaining successful fusion and good clinical results. If patients exhibit minimal or no deformity, the ankle fusion can be done through an arthroscope or a minimally invasive "mini-open" technique. These basic fusion procedures may not be as effective in patients who have adjacent joint arthritis or increasing bone loss and deformity. Other patient factors such as diabetes, Charcot neuroarthropathy, and infection also may render ankle arthritis more difficult to manage. The treating surgeon must adapt to address more complex types of ankle arthritis effectively by performing a TTC, pantalar, or TC fusion rather than a strict ankle joint fusion. Certain patient circumstances require the use of external fixation, which can be more challenging to use than internal fixation.

Finally, the role of ankle arthrodesis recently has expanded as a means to salvage a patient's limb. The circumstances that bring a patient to require such a procedure also can be complex.

Ankle arthrodesis is by no means a simple surgery. It requires preoperative planning, meticulous preparation of bony surfaces, cognizance of ankle positioning, and rigidity of fixation. The procedure also requires enough experience on the part of the operating surgeon to recognize important patient factors and to assess which type of ankle arthrodesis is most appropriate for that specific patient.

References

[1] Raikin S. Arthrodesis of the ankle: arthroscopic, mini-open, and open techniques. Foot Ankle Clin 2003;8:347–59.

[2] Thomas R, Daniels T. Ankle arthritis. J Bone Joint Surg Am 2003;85:923–36.

[3] Albert E. Beitrage zur operativen chiurgie. Zur resection des kniegelenkes. Wien Med Press 1879;20:705–8.

[4] Demetriades L, Strauss E, Gallina J. Osteoarthritis of the ankle. Clin Orthop Relat Res 1998; 349:48–57.

[5] Buck P, Morrey B, Chao E. The optimum position of arthrodesis of the ankle. A gait study of the knee and ankle. J Bone Joint Surg Am 1987;69:1052–62.

[6] Mann R, Van Manen J, Wapner K. Ankle fusion. Clin Orthop Relat Res 1991;268: 49–55.

[7] Flackiger G, Weber M. The transfibular approach for ankle arthrodesis. Oper Orthop Traumatol 2005;17(4–5):361–79.

[8] Grass R, Rammelt S, Biewener A, et al. Arthrodesis of the ankle joint. Clin Podiatr Med Surg 2004;21(2):161–78.

[9] Dohm M, Benjamin J, Harrison J. A biomechanical evaluation of three forms of internal fixation used in ankle arthrodesis. Foot Ankle Int 1994;15:297–300.

[10] Ogilvie-Harris D, Fitsialos D, Hedman T. Arthrodesis of the ankle. A comparison of two versus three screw fixation in a crossed configuration. Clin Orthop Relat Res 1994;304:195–9.

[11] Verkelst M, Mulier J, Hoogmartens M. Arthrodesis of the ankle joint with complete removal of the distal part of the fibula: experience with the transfibular approach and three different types of fixation. Clin Orthop Relat Res 1976;118:93–9.

[12] Holt E, Hansen S, Mayo K. Ankle arthrodesis using internal screw fixation. Clin Orthop Relat Res 1991;268:21–8.

[13] Nasson S, Shuff C, Palmer D, et al. Biomechanical comparison of ankle arthrodesis techniques: crossed screws vs. blade plate. Foot Ankle Int 2001;22(7):575–80.

[14] Mann R, Rongstad K. Arthrodesis of the ankle: a critical analysis. Foot Ankle Int 1998; 19(1):3–9.

[15] Colman A, Pomeroy G. Transfibular ankle arthrodesis with rigid internal fixation: an assessment of outcome. Foot Ankle Int 2007;28(3):303–7.

[16] Abidi N, Gruen G, Conti S. Ankle arthrodesis: indications and techniques. J Am Acad Orthop Surg 2000;8(3):200–9.

[17] Klaue K, Bursic D. The dorsolateral approach to the ankle for arthrodesis. Oper Orthop Traumatol 2005;17(4–5):380–91.

[18] Scranton P. Use of internal compression in arthrodesis of the ankle. J Bone Joint Surg Am 1985;67(4):550–5.

[19] Marcus R, Balourdas G, Heiple K. Ankle arthrodesis by chevron fusion with internal fixation and bone-grafting. J Bone Joint Surg Am 1983;65(6):833–8.

[20] Eylon S, Porat S, Bor N, et al. Outcome of Ilizarov ankle arthrodesis. Foot Ankle Int 2007; 28(8):873–9.

[21] Labitzke R. Ankle arthrodesis using the cable technique. Oper Orthop Traumatol 2005; 17(4–5):392–406.

[22] Mackley T, Schatz T, Srivastava S, et al. [Ankle arthrodesis with intramedullary compression nailing]. Unfallchirurg 2003;106(9):732–40 [in German].

[23] Tarkin I, Mormino M, Clare M, et al. Anterior plate supplementation increases ankle arthrodesis construct rigidity. Foot Ankle Int 2007;28(2):219–23.

[24] Schneider D. Arthroscopic surgery of the ankle, arthroscopic abrasion arthroplasty, ankle fusion. Arthroscopy Video Journal 1983;3(2):35–47.

[25] Morgan C. Arthroscopic tibio-talar arthrodesis. The Jefferson Orthopaedic Journal 1987;16: 50–2.

[26] Myerson M, Allon S. Arthroscopic ankle arthrodesis. Contemp Orthop 1989;19:21–7.

[27] Ogilvie-Harris D, Lieberman I, Fitsialos D. Arthroscopically assisted arthrodesis for osteoarthrotic ankles. J Bone Joint Surg Am 1993;75:1167–73.

[28] Zvijac J, Lemak L, Schurhoff M, et al. Analysis of arthroscopically assisted ankle arthrodesis. Arthroscopy 2002;18(1):70–5.

[29] Myerson M, Quill G. Ankle arthrodesis: a comparison of an arthroscopic and an open method of treatment. Clin Orthop Relat Res 1991;268:84–95.

[30] Winson I, Robinson D, Allen P. Arthroscopic ankle arthrodesis. J Bone Joint Surg Br 2005; 87(3):343–7.

[31] Paremain G, Miller S, Myerson M. Ankle arthrodesis: results after the miniarthrotomy technique. Foot Ankle Int 1996;17(5):247–52.

[32] Miller S, Paremain G, Myerson M. The miniarthrotomy technique of ankle arthrodesis: a cadaver study of operative vascular compromise and early clinical results. Orthopedics 1996; 19(5):425–30.

[33] Gruen G, Mears D. Arthrodesis of the ankle and subtalar joints. Clin Orthop Relat Res 1991;268:15–20.

[34] Haddad S, Mann R. Flatfoot deformity in adults. In: Coughlin M, Mann R, Saltzman C, editors. Surgery of the foot and ankle. 8th edition. Philadelphia: Mosby Elsevier; 2007. p. 1007–86.

[35] Kelly I, Easley M. Treatment of stage 3 adult acquired flatfoot. Foot Ankle Clin 2001;6(1): 153–66.

[36] Bohay D, Anderson J. Stage IV posterior tibial tendon insufficiency: the tilted ankle. Foot Ankle Clin 2003;8(3):619–36.

[37] Kelly I, Nunley J. Treatment of stage 4 adult acquired flatfoot. Foot Ankle Clin 2001;6(1): 167–78.

[38] Faillace J, Leopold S, Brage M. Extended hindfoot fusions and pantalar fusions—history, biomechanics, and clinical results. Foot Ankle Clin 2000;5(4):777–98.

[39] Saltzman C. Ankle arthritis. In: Coughlin M, Mann R, Saltzman C, editors. Surgery of the foot and ankle. 8th edition. Philadelphia: Mosby Elsevier; 2007. p. 923–83.

[40] Mendicino R, Catanzariti A, Saltrick K, et al. Tibiotalocalcaneal arthrodesis with retrograde intramedullary nailing. J Foot Ankle Surg 2004;43(2):82–6.

[41] Quill G. Tibiotalocalcaneal and pantalar arthrodesis. Foot Ankle Clin 1996;1:199–209.

[42] Quill G. Tibiotalocalcaneal arthrodesis. Tech Orthop 1996;11:269–73.

[43] Russotti G, Johnson K, Cass J. Tibiotalocalcaneal arthrodesis for arthritis and deformity of the hind part of the foot. J Bone Joint Surg Am 1988;70:1304–7.

[44] Kile T, Donnelly R, Gehrke J, et al. Tibiotalocalcaneal arthrodesis with an intramedullary device. Foot Ankle Int 1994;15:669–73.

[45] Chou L, Mann R, Yaszay B, et al. Tibiotalocalcaneal arthrodesis. Foot Ankle Int 2000; 21(10):804–8.

[46] Chiodo C, Acevedo J, Sammarco V, et al. Intramedullary rod fixation compared with blade-plate-and-screw fixation for tibiotalocalcaneal arthrodesis: a biomechanical investigation. J Bone Joint Surg Am 2003;85(12):2425–8.

[47] Hanson T, Cracchiolo A. The use of a 95 degree blade plate and a posterior approach to achieve tibiotalocalcaneal arthrodesis. Foot Ankle Int 2002;23(8):704–10.

[48] Acosta R, Ushiba J, Cracchiolo A. The results of a primary and staged pantalar arthrodesis and tibiotalocalcaneal arthrodesis in adult patients. Foot Ankle Int 2000;21(3):182–94.

[49] Ahmad J, Eslam Pour A, Raikin S. The modified use of a proximal humerus locking plate for tibiotalocalcaneal arthrodesis. Foot Ankle Int 2007;28(9):977–83.

[50] Muir D, Angliss R, Nattrass G, et al. Tibiotalocalcaneal arthrodesis for severe calcaneovalgus deformity in cerebral palsy. J Pediatr Orthop 2005;25(5):651–6.

[51] Mann R. Arthrodesis of the foot and ankle. In: Coughlin M, Mann R, Saltzman C, editors. Surgery of the foot and ankle. 8th edition. Philadelphia: Mosby Elsevier; 2007. p. 1087–123.

[52] Papa J, Myerson M. Pantalar and tibiotalocalcaneal arthrodesis for post-traumatic osteoarthrosis of the ankle and hindfoot. J Bone Joint Surg Am 1992;74:1042–9.

[53] Mulfinger GL, Trueta J. The blood supply of the talus. J Bone Joint Surg Br 1970;52:160–7.

[54] Peterson L, Goldie I, Lindell D. The arterial supply of the talus. Acta Orthop Scand 1974;45: 260–70.

[55] Peterson L, Goldie I. The arterial supply of the talus: a study on the relationship to experimental talus fractures. Acta Orthop Scand 1975;46:1026–34.

[56] Horst F, Gilbert B, Nunley J. Avascular necrosis of the talus: current treatment options. Foot Ankle Clin 2004;9:757–73.

[57] Mindell E, Cisek E, Kartalian G. Late results of injuries to the talus: analysis of forty cases. J Bone Joint Surg Am 1963;45:221–45.

[58] Canale S, Kelly FB Jr. Fractures of the neck of the talus: long-term evaluation of seventy-one cases. J Bone Joint Surg Am 1978;60:143–56.

[59] Mont M, Schon L, Hungerford MW, et al. Avascular necrosis of the talus treated by core decompression. J Bone Joint Surg Br 1996;78:827–30.

[60] Hussl H, Sialer R, Daniaux H, et al. Revascularization of a partially necrotic talus with a vascularized bone graft from the iliac crest. Arch Orthop Trauma Surg 1989;108:27–9.

[61] Blair H. Comminuted fractures and fracture dislocations of the body of the astragalus. Operative treatment. Am J Surg 1943;59:37–43.

[62] Morris H. Aseptic necrosis of the talus following injury. Orthop Clin North Am 1974;5: 166–89.

[63] Dennis M, Tullos H. Blair tibiotalar arthrodesis for injuries to the talus. J Bone Joint Surg Am 1980;62:103–7.

[64] Van Bergeyk A, Stotler W, Beals T, et al. Functional outcome after modified Blair tibiotalar arthrodesis for talar osteonecrosis. Foot Ankle Int 2003;24(10):765–70.

[65] Kitoaka H, Patzer G. Arthrodesis for the treatment of arthrodesis of the ankle and osteonecrosis of the talus. J Bone Joint Surg Am 1998;80:370–9.

[66] Adelaar R, Madrian J. Avascular necrosis of the talus. Orthop Clin North Am 2004;35(3): 385–95.

[67] Joseph T, Myerson M. Use of talectomy in modern foot and ankle surgery. Foot Ankle Clin North Am 2004;9:775–85.

[68] Mann R, Chou L. Tibiocalcaneal arthrodesis. Foot Ankle Int 1995;16(7):401–5.

[69] Myerson M, Alavarez R, Lam P. Tibiocalcaneal arthrodesis for the management of severe ankle and hindfoot deformities. Foot Ankle Int 2000;21(8):643–50.

[70] Dennison M, Pool RD, Simonis RB. Tibiocalcaneal fusion for avascular necrosis of the talus. J Bone Joint Surg Br 2001;83(2):199–203.

[71] Baumhauer J, Lu A, DiGiovanni B. Arthodesis of the infected ankle and subtalar joint. Foot Ankle Clin 2002;7(1):175–90.

[72] Kollig E, Esenwein S, Muhr G, et al. Fusion of the septic ankle: experience with 15 cases using hybrid external fixation. J Trauma 2003;55(4):685–91.

[73] Saltzman C. Salvage of diffuse ankle osteomyelitis by single-stage resection and circumferential frame compression arthrodesis. Iowa Orthop J 2005;25:47–52.

[74] Kolker D, Wilson M. Tibiocalcaneal arthrodesis after total talectomy for treatment of osteomyelitis of the talus. Foot Ankle Int 2004;25(12):861–5.

[75] Thordarson D, Patzakis M, Holtom P, et al. Salvage of the septic ankle with concomitant tibial osteomyelitis. Foot Ankle Int 1997;18(3):151–6.

[76] Caravaggi C, Cimmino M, Caruso S, et al. Intramedullary compressive nail fixation for the treatment of severe Charcot deformity of the ankle and rear foot. J Foot Ankle Surg 2006; 45(1):20–4.

[77] Dalla Paola L, Volpe A, Varotto D, et al. Use of a retrograde nail for ankle arthrodesis in Charcot neuroarthropathy: a limb salvage procedure. Foot Ankle Int 2007;28(9):967–70.

[78] Cooper P. Application of external fixators for management of Charcot deformities of the foot and ankle. Foot Ankle Clin 2002;7(1):207–54.

[79] Herbst S. External fixation of Charcot arthropathy. Foot Ankle Clin 2004;9:595–609.

[80] Fabrin J, Larsen K, Holstein P. Arthrodesis with external fixation in the unstable or misaligned Charcot ankle in patients with diabetes mellitus. Int J Low Extrem Wounds 2007; 6(2):102–7.

[81] Pinzur M, Noonan T. Ankle arthrodesis with a retrograde femoral nail for Charcot ankle arthropathy. Foot Ankle Int 2005;26(7):545–9.

[82] Hockenbury R, Gruttadauria M, McKinney I. Use of implantable bone growth stimulation in Charcot ankle arthrodesis. Foot Ankle Int 2007;28(9):971–6.

[83] Haddad S, Coetzee J, Estok R, et al. Intermediate and long-term outcomes of total ankle arthroplasty and ankle arthrodesis. A systematic review of the literature. J Bone Joint Surg Am 2007;89:1899–905.

[84] Stamatis E, Myerson M. How to avoid specific complications of total ankle replacement. Foot Ankle Clin 2002;7(4):765–89.

[85] Myerson M, Miller S. Salvage after complications of total ankle arthroplasty. Foot Ankle Clin 2002;7(1):191–206.

[86] Conti S, Wong Y. Complications of total ankle replacement. Foot Ankle Clin 2002;7(4): 791–807.

[87] Wapner K. Salvage of failed and infected total ankle replacements with fusion. Instr Course Lect 2002;51:153–7.

[88] Zarutsky E, Rush S, Schuberth J. The use of circular wire external fixation in the treatment of salvage ankle arthrodesis. J Foot Ankle Surg 2005;44(1):22–31.

[89] Carlsson A, Montgomery F, Besjakov J. Arthrodesis of the ankle secondary to replacement. Foot Ankle Int 1998;19(4):240–5.

[90] Gabrion A, Jarda O, Havet E, et al. [Ankle arthrodesis after failure of a total ankle prosthesis. Eight cases]. Revue de chirurgie orthopedique et reparatrice de l'appareil moteur 2004; 90(4):353–9 [in French].

[91] Hopgood P, Kumar R, Wood P. Ankle arthrodesis for failed total ankle replacement. J Bone Joint Surg Br 2006;88(8):1032–8.

[92] Culpan P, Le Strat V, Piriou P, et al. Arthrodesis after failed total ankle replacement. J Bone Joint Surg Br 2007;89:1178–83.

[93] Johl C, Kircher J, Pohlmannn K, et al. Management of failed total ankle replacement with a retrograde short femoral nail: a case report. J Orthop Trauma 2006;20(1):60–5.

[94] Schill S. Ankle arthrodesis with interposition graft as a salvage procedure after failed total ankle replacement. Oper Orthop Traumatol 2007;19(5–6):547–60.

[95] Castro J, Hernandez M, Sierra A, et al. Distal tibial reconstruction and ankle arthrodesis in osteosarcoma (salvage technique). A case presentation. Acta Ortop Mex 2007;21(5):289–95.

[96] Moore D, Halpern J, Schwartz H. Allograft ankle arthrodesis: a limb salvage technique for distal tibial tumors. Clin Orthop Relat Res 2005;440:213–21.

[97] Hiraizumi Y, Hara T, Takahashi M, et al. Open total dislocation of the talus with extrusion (missing talus): report of two cases. Foot Ankle Int 1992;13(8):473–7.

[98] Koller H, Assuncao A, Kolb K, et al. Reconstructive surgery for complete talus extrusion using the sandwich block arthrodesis: a report of 2 cases. J Foot Ankle Surg 2007;46(6): 493–8.

ELSEVIER
SAUNDERS

Foot Ankle Clin N Am
13 (2008) 401–416

FOOT AND
ANKLE CLINICS

An Approach to the Failed Ankle Arthrodesis

Steven M. Raikin, MD[a,b],*, Venkat Rampuri, MD[a]

[a]Orthopaedic Surgery, Jefferson Medical College, Thomas Jefferson University Hospital,
111 S. 11th street, Philadelphia, PA 19107, USA
[b]Orthopaedic Foot and Ankle Service, Rothman Institute, 925 Chestnut Street, Philadelphia,
PA 19107, USA

Ankle arthrodesis has been used successfully for end-stage arthritis of the ankle for more than a century [1]. It has proved to be successful in relieving pain by eliminating motion and providing stability with a well-aligned plantigrade foot [2–8]. Arthrodesis has remained the gold standard for end-stage posttraumatic arthritis, against which other surgical procedures for ankle arthritis are compared for clinical and functional benefits [9,10]. Originally devised for poliomyelitis and tuberculosis of the ankle, the indications for ankle arthrodesis have changed over time. Current indications include isolated end-stage arthritis from a posttraumatic, postinfective, avascular necrosis or an inflammatory etiology. Fusion of a Charcot neuropathy of the ankle was previously avoided because of the high incidence of nonunion; however, recent studies seem to show with the current improved methods of fusion that it is a reasonable option [11–13].

Fusion rates ranging from 80% to 100% have been reported in the literature [7], along with patient satisfaction rates of more than 80% [14]. Intermediate and long-term studies have shown functional deterioration over time, however [2–8]. Successful outcome often depends on the reason for which the fusion was performed. Patients who undergo ankle arthrodesis after a bacterial infection or neuropathic ankle arthropathy often have poor results in comparison to other causes [15,16]. Unrecognized involvement of adjacent joints in the arthritic process may lead to persistent pain despite successful fusion; it should be evaluated before surgery with careful radiologic assessment or be treated with selective joint injections.

* Orthopaedic Surgery, Jefferson Medical College, Thomas Jefferson University Hospital, 111 S. 11th Street, Philadelphia, PA 19107.
    E-mail address: steven.raikin@rothmaninstitute.com (S.M. Raikin).

1083-7515/08/$ - see front matter © 2008 Elsevier Inc. All rights reserved.
doi:10.1016/j.fcl.2008.04.009

Detailed gait analysis after an ankle arthrodesis has shown decreased cadence and stride length with decreased range of motion of the hind foot and midfoot during the stance and swing phases of the gait [8]. This loss of motion deteriorates further with development of subtalar and midfoot arthritis [8,15], which leads to long-term failure. It is important to recognize that in light of its success and failures, ankle arthrodesis is a salvage option in patients with pain and stiffness [17].

The study by Said and colleagues [18] found that all their failed ankle fusions required revision surgeries; however, reoperation rates for failed fusions have been quoted to range from 50% to 70% [14,19]. Complications of ankle arthrodesis could be categorized broadly into early or short-term, intermediate, and long-term and include wound-related complications, neurovascular injuries, infections, malunions from malpositioning, non-unions, adjacent joint arthritis, limb shortening, and limb atrophy. This article reviews various complications of the open arthrodesis procedures and discusses the potential causes of these problems. It also addresses their prevention and the options of management of these often difficult problems.

Short-term complications

Postoperative recuperation after a successful ankle arthrodesis includes a long rehabilitation process, with most people returning to early activities on average 12 months after the fusion [14]. Short-term or early complications could be defined as complications that occur from the immediate postoperative period to the first 6 months after surgery. Early complications predominantly involve wound-related problems and infections. Other associated complications, such as nerve injury, complex regional pain syndrome, deep venous thrombosis, pulmonary embolism, and other medical problems, in the early postoperative period also can delay a successful rehabilitation.

Wound-related problems

Wound-related complications seem to be in direct relation to the surgical technique and handling of soft tissues during the surgery. Many patients have had prior surgery, with multiple scars and adhesions within the soft tissue envelope around the ankle. The surgeon should attempt to use prior incisions when possible and create adequate thickness of the skin flaps to optimize vascular supply to the skin edges. When it is not possible to use a prior incision, care should be taken to ensure adequate angiosomal circulation to the skin bridge between incisions to prevent necrosis and breakdown, which can lead to infection.

Most wound problems involve delayed wound healing or a superficial wound infection. Superficial infection of the surgical incision or the pin sites in external fixation methods has been reported as occurring in 40% to 50%

of cases [5,20–23]. Most of these infections do not cause long-term morbidity but need to be managed with care. Prophylactic measures, such as preoperative antibiotics, a meticulous sterile surgical technique, and prevention of excessive traction of skin, help to prevent these problems. Unless infection is present, antibiotics should not be started and local wound care usually suffices. In the presence of a superficial infection, a broad-spectrum oral antibiotic may suffice together with dressing changes. Superficial wound cultures are controversial because of high contamination rates but may be useful in directing antibiotic selection.

It is important to recognize high-risk patients, such as patients with dysvascular skin, rheumatoid arthritis, or diabetes, patients on long-term steroids, and patients undergoing revision surgeries. If treated early, these superficial wound infections tend to heal well without further problems; a delay in recognizing these infections could result in disastrous results, such as amputation [18].

Deep infection

Deep infections after ankle fusion could lead to deep sepsis and osteomyelitis, with disastrous consequences [18]. Recognition of such conditions is essential because they are not amenable to simple oral antibiotics. A thorough surgical irrigation and debridement of the wound combined with an adequate (usually 6-week) course of intravenous antibiotics is necessary to treat the infection. If the infection involves the internal hardware, removal followed by stabilization with an external fixation device can salvage the arthrodesis and allow successful fusion to occur [24]. The remaining wound may not be able to be closed primarily and should be managed with vacuum-assisted secondary closure or application of a myocutaneous flap [25]. The rate of amputation in patients with persistent osteomyelitis and an ongoing infection with drainage despite these measures could be as high as 50% [18,20,23,26], which happens more so in the case of fusions performed in the face of an existing septic process.

Intermediate-term complications

Intermediate-term complications could be defined as complications that occur between the first 6 months and 1 year after the fusion. During this period, the fusion is consolidated into a bony construct, which allows patients to progressively increase their weight-bearing status and return to their activities. Malunions caused by malpositioning and nonunion are the two major complications during this period. Other minor complications during this period include chronic edema, stress fractures, and calluses.

The ideal position in which the ankle is fused has changed over time [27]. Previously the ankle was fused in a more equinus position to allow patients to wear shoes with heels. This approach has been discontinued because gait studies demonstrated a vaulting gait pattern with a recurvatum thrust at the knee [3,28]. The currently accepted position for fusion involves the ankle being held in neutral dorsiflexion/plantar flexion, 5° of valgus, 5° to 10° of external rotation, and slightly posteriorly displaced talus relative to the tibia [3,27]. The overall alignment of foot to the rest of limb should be assessed and compared with the opposite side before accepting the fusion. In a gait analysis conducted by Mazur and colleagues [3], this position was shown to produce a more normal pattern of gait and decrease the stress around the knee. Posterior placement of the talus under the tibia has been described to reduce the anterior lever arm of the foot under the arthrodesis. Although anterior placement, which can cause difficulties with the foot clearing the ground during swing phase of the gait, should be avoided, the theoretic advantage of posterior placement has not proved to be clinically relevant.

Malunions

Sagittal plane deformities

Variations from the accepted positions of alignment could be labeled as malunions or malpositions. Excessive dorsiflexion or plantar flexion beyond plantigrade position could transform into flexion or extension deformities of the knee leading to gait disturbances. An ankle fused in an equinus position results in a vaulting gait secondary to the recurvatum deformity at the knee (Fig. 1), which occurs as a compensatory mechanism by which

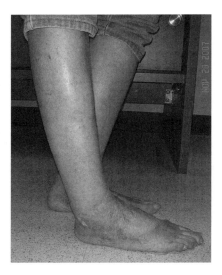

Fig. 1. Clinical picture of a patient whose ankle has been fused in equinus. Note the recuvatum of the knee required to allow the foot to be plantargrade on the floor.

the patient clears the foot off the ground during the gait cycle. Such a pathologic gait puts undue stress not only across the knee but also at the anterior tibia and the midfoot, which results in stress fractures and metatarsalgia. Alternately, patients may externally rotate their leg while walking, which puts increased stress on the medial aspect of the knee and the hind foot. Treatment of a symptomatic equinus deformity starts with the use of a solid ankle cushion heel shoe to improve mechanics and alleviate symptoms. Surgery is offered to patients who remain symptomatic despite these measures.

Fusion of the ankle in a dorsiflexed position results in increased pressure on the heel pad, which causes pain and potential breakdown. Gait alterations include ambulating with a flexed knee to maintain a plantigrade foot, which can be corrected by using a rocker bottom sole shoe, with surgery being indicated in recalcitrant cases.

Revision surgery for sagittal plane deformities involves realignment osteotomies through the fusion mass, which can be done through closing wedge or opening wedge realignment procedures, with closing wedge osteotomies being more frequently used. They diminish stretch to associated nerves and the soft tissue and allow bone-to-bone approximation with high fusion rates. The disadvantage, however, is that further limb shortening occurs as a result of the bony resection from the osteotomy site. Dome-shaped osteotomies are technically more challenging but are less likely to affect limb length. Correction of an equinus deformity involves either a posterior opening wedge or an anterior closing wedge osteotomy (Fig. 2), whereas dorsiflexion malunion can be corrected with either an anterior opening or a posterior closing wedge osteotomy. Determination of the approach often lies with several factors, such as prior incisions and associated leg length discrepancies. The amount of bone to be resected and the place of resection often need to be individualized from patient to patient.

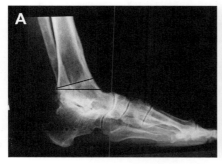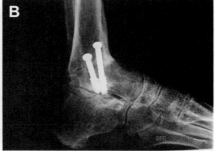

Fig. 2. (*A*) Lateral radiograph of the ankle fused in equinus. Lines are drawn to represent the planned corrective anterior closing wedge osteotomy. The proximal osteotomy cut is perpendicular to the long axis of the tibia, whereas the distal cut is parallel to the floor. (*B*) Lateral radiograph shows final correction after successful osteotomy and revision arthrodesis with ankle in neutral alignment.

Coronal plane deformities

Positioning of the ankle fusion in more than 5° of valgus or any degree of varus can cause undue stresses across the hind foot (Fig. 3) and the knee. An excessive valgus position causes undue stress on the posterior tibial tendon and the ligamentous structures on the medial aspect of the ankle, which results in development of a flat foot posture. These forces could transmit proximally and stress the inner aspect of the knee. Walking on a foot aligned in excess valgus also puts undue stress on the medial column and the first tarsometatarsal joint complex, which results in stress fractures or premature arthritis in this area. Initial use of medial hind foot wedge orthotic inserts to tilt the foot into varus should be attempted. Failure requires surgical correction using a medial closing wedge osteotomy of the fusion mass. A transfibular approach with a lateral wedge is also an option if the prior incisions dictate the approach.

No degree of varus alignment is tolerated after arthrodesis of the ankle joint, which results in undue stress on the subtalar joint and the peroneal tendons, lateral ligamentous structures, and lateral column of the foot. This stress eventually may result in stress fractures of the fifth metatarsal bone, premature subtalar joint arthritis, or peroneal tendon pathology. Initial treatment involves an orthotic insert with a lateral posting to drive the foot into a neutral position, which can be combined with a lateral flare to redistribute the pressure on the bottom of the foot. Surgical management includes a lateral closing wedge osteotomy of the fusion mass to correct the deformity.

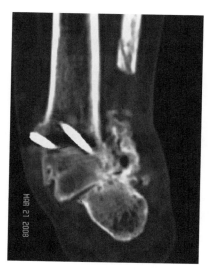

Fig. 3. CT scan of an ankle fused in valgus, with subsequent lateral subluxation and secondary valgus arthritis of the subtalar joint of the hindfoot.

Chronic deformity results in secondary changes in the hind foot and fore-foot alignment. Many patients require additional bony and soft tissue procedures around the foot so as to obtain a well-aligned plantar grade foot after realignment osteotomy. Correction of any associated rotational elements is also feasible with this approach.

Rotational and complex deformities

Excess internal or external rotation of the foot in relation to the tibia could lead to a compensatory torsional defect of the tibia and result in undue torsional stress on the knee. Rotation deformities often are associated with some other planar deformities and often require adequate surgical planning. Although most of these malpositions or malalignments can be diagnosed by sheer clinical examination, it is essential to do a gait analysis along with a CT scan comparison to the unaffected side to assess the alignment before a revision surgery is undertaken for these patients. These scans help in identifying the direction of malunions, because it often could be multiplanar instead of isolated sagittal or coronal planar deformity. Correction of multiplanar deformities may require multiplanar osteotomies and often are complex to perform. They may be best corrected by external devices such as an Ilizarov or a Taylor spatial frame (Smith and Nephew, Memphis, TN) type of construct. Recently, conversion to a total ankle replacement has been shown to relieve symptoms of ankle fusion malunions while obtaining correction of the deformity [29]. The long-term efficacy of these procedures is unknown, however, and amputation rates of 13% have been reported [29].

Nonunions

With improving methods of fixation, rates of unions are also improving; however, nonunion still remains one of the leading causes of failures [30]. Fusion usually occurs within 3 months of surgery, with delayed union defined as taking 3 to 6 months and nonunions taking more than 6 months to fuse. Delayed union seen radiographically or suggested by persistent weight-bearing pain in the ankle region is managed by prolonged periods of immobilization and protected weight bearing. The addition of an external bone stimulator can be used to promote maturation of the fusion mass and advance the fusion.

Nonunions of the ankle arthrodesis are often painful and require corrective revision surgery. Although there are several risk factors for nonunion, one of the leading causes is the cause for which the fusion was performed. A recent meta-analysis described a nonunion rate of 10%, with 65% of revision surgeries performed on failed ankle fusion being done to treat nonunions [31]. Historically, nonunion rates have been reported to occur from less than 5% [3,14,31,32] to 41% [26,33]; however, with current improved methods of fixation the union rates have improved to more than 90% [34,35]. Preoperative infection [36], sensory neuropathy [19,22,37], and avascular necrosis of the talus [38] seem to be affected with higher rates of nonunion (as high as 100%).

Among patients with posttraumatic arthritis, high-energy fractures that result in talar dome fractures [38,39] and tibial plafond fractures [20,38] and those with open fractures also have higher rates of nonunion. Other historical risk factors associated with nonunions include a history of diabetes or renal disease or other major medical comorbidities [38], history of smoking tobacco [40,41], rheumatoid arthritis [42], psychiatric ailment [42], and a previous history of subtalar arthrodesis [43]. Other intraoperative factors, such as strength and method of fixation, bone defects and bone loss, poor bony apposition, and bony preparation during fixation, could result in failures [42]. Similarly, postoperative factors, such as inadequate immobilization after surgery and poor compliance, also could adversely affect union rates.

Approach to nonunions

Treatment of a nonunion depends on the symptoms that a patient experiences. Revision surgery is indicated only in patients with a painful nonunion. A nonunion in a patient with neuropathy, if stable and asymptomatic, is often best treated with bracing [44]. Most nonunions ultimately require revision surgery, however.

Accurate identification and diagnosis of the cause behind a nonunion are essential before revision surgery is undertaken. Although a certain percentage of nonunions occurs without a definitive underlying cause, a potential cause always should be excluded and reversed before revision surgery. Nonunion usually occurs as a result of inadequate surgical technique at the index procedure (poor joint preparation or inadequate fixation), an inadequate healing milieu, or an infection. The process of critical analysis begins with a thorough history and physical examination, including a review of the previous surgical procedure. If the nonunion is a result of a poor surgical technique (Fig. 4), it may be easiest to revise with a takedown on the nonunion, appropriate joint preparation, bone grafting, and rigid fixation.

Patient-associated risk factors can influence the healing environment and increase the risk of nonunion. Although some factors, such as age and neuroarthropathy, cannot be altered, a surgeon should assess and correct all factors that can be improved. Cigarette smoking is a leading cause of fusion nonunions [40], and patients should be convinced to discontinue smoking before undertaking any revision surgery. Newer medications, such as varenicline (Chantix), together with counseling can assist patients with their cessation program without the continued use of nicotine infused through traditional patches and gums. Although there is no evidence whether temporary smoking cessation prevents nonunion, it is anecdotally felt that discontinuation of cigarette smoking at least 1 to 2 weeks before surgery (and continued after surgery) may improve microcirculation. On a similar note, patients who have rheumatoid arthritis are also advised to withhold

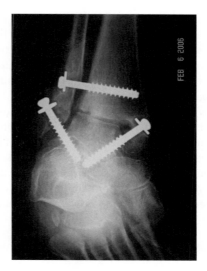

Fig. 4. Anteroposterior radiograph demonstrates inadequate joint preparation and fixation, resulting in this nonunion of an ankle fusion 9 months after surgery.

immunosuppressant medication for 2 weeks before and 2 weeks after surgery, despite literature supporting the fact that these medications do not increase the risk of nonunions or infections [45].

Patients who have diabetes should be counseled on the importance of normal blood sugar levels before and after the surgery because they has a direct bearing on the union. Patients with comorbidities should be optimized by their medical team before revision surgery is undertaken. Nutrition should be optimized, and a prealbumin level of more than 18 mg/dL is preferable before surgery is undertaken. In the absence of infection or osteonecrosis, once these factors are corrected, a standard-type revision arthrodesis can be undertaken. This procedure is performed with minimal soft tissue stripping, removal of all fibrous tissue from the nonunion site down to bleeding trabecular bone, use of autologous or allograft type of bone grafting, and appropriate rigid fixation. Strict adherence to compliance with postoperative restrictions must be reinforced and adhered to, including restricted weight bearing and external support until full consolidation occurs, which may take 4 to 6 months. Internal or external bone stimulation has not been found to be useful in an established nonunion but may be useful after revision surgery [46].

An ankle nonunion that swells up with erythema and is warm to touch is an infective nonunion until proven otherwise. Investigation of an infected nonunion starts with a serologic evaluation, including a complete blood count, erythrocyte sedimentation rate, and a C-reactive protein. Although elevated erythrocyte sedimentation rate and C-reactive protein levels are not diagnostic themselves, they are important indicators of infection and can be useful baselines in monitoring treatment. Aspiration of nonunion is diagnostic in only 50% to 60% of cases [47]; however, it is the most specific test that yields direct information, which helps manage these conditions. Imaging studies are often not specific enough to elucidate the cause of nonunion but form an important part in presurgical planning. Radiologic studies often begin with a series of weight-bearing radiographs that are often supplemented by a CT scan to look for osseous defects. A contrast-enhanced MRI scan sometimes may be useful in identifying osteonecrosis of the talus as an origin of the nonunion. Nuclear scans are often misused; however, a negative technetium bone scan result can help rule out septic nonunion (although it often demonstrates increased activity in any nonunion and is poorly specific for infection). [111]In or Ceretec-labeled white blood infusion scans have a higher specificity in diagnosing infected nonunions.

Confirmed infected nonunions require surgical management. In most cases they require a staged correction [48–51], which first eliminates the infection and subsequently treats the nonunion. This approach involves an initial removal of hardware, together with resection of all the infected pseudoarthrosis tissue along with debridement of the nonviable sclerotic osseous elements. Remaining defects are filled with antibiotic-impregnated bone cement beads; a course of intravenous organism-specific antibiotic management is initiated and usually continues for at least 6 weeks. The second procedure is performed once the infection has been eradicated. If uncertainty persists, a frozen section biopsy can be taken at the second surgery and evaluated before insertion of internal fixation. If the result is positive, repeat debridement, irrigation, and antibiotic cement bead insertion are performed. If the infection has been eradicated, bone grafting and filling all the osseous defects during the second stage are important to provide adequate fixation and stimulus for a union.

The type of fixation required to achieve this could be either external or internal. Although no prospective randomized controlled trials have compared the two methods, there is an inclination for external fixators, because they avoid placement of any foreign material at the site of fusion [52]. External fixation could be in the form of a circular skinny wire type frame (Fig. 5) or other unilateral or triangular frames constructs placed with compression across the joint area. External fixators offer some other advantages, such as ease of caring for wound and soft-tissue– related problems, ability to correct three-dimensional deformities (including limb length inequalities), and ability to bear weight early [24]. Potential problems and difficulties include pin tract infections, knee contractures or stiffness, and secondary surgery for removal of the frame [24]. When the bone stock is adequate for a good internal fixation, fusion using large cannulated screws in a cross-screw fashion with bone grafting could be attempted. This fixation could be supplemented by either a rigid plating device or an external fixation for additional support and stability. Such choices often depend on the intra-operative stability as assessed by the surgeon and the exposure required for the revision. An alternative approach is to perform a one-stage procedure

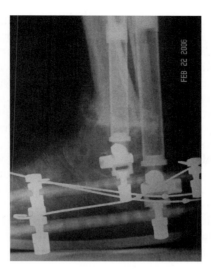

Fig. 5. Lateral radiograph demonstrates a successful revision fusion of an infected nonunion of a prior attempted arthrodesis using a skinny wire-type external fixator device.

with extensive debridement of infected and nonviable tissue followed by the immediate application of a compression external fixation device. Patients who have had multiple revision surgeries for septic nonunion are sometimes better off with a below-knee amputation and a prosthesis, especially when the bone loss is substantive [29].

An additional cause of aseptic nonunion of ankle arthrodesis is talar osteonecrosis. Revision surgery may require large portions of the talus to be removed until viable healing surfaces are obtained. These patients often fare better with other salvage procedures, such as tibiotalocalcaneal arthrodesis or tibiocalcaneal arthrodesis. Autologous bone graft supplementation and augmenting bone stimulators may increase the fusion rate of these procedures. Kitaoka and Patzer [53] reported on 19 patients who underwent this procedure. They reported a fusion rate of 84% (16/19), but only 68% of patients rated their results as good or excellent. Although both of these procedures can be performed either as open procedures with rigid internal fixation methods by cross-screw technique or rigid plating, recent studies have been shown to achieve comparable results with lower complication rates using retrograde nailing [54].

Long-term complications

Adjacent joint arthritis

Adjacent segment disease after fusion is a well-proven and well-documented entity in the spinal literature. In their long-term follow-up study,

Coester and colleagues [6] showed that after a mean follow-up period of 22 years after an ankle arthrodesis, all patients had radiographic features in the surrounding joints that suggested degenerative arthritis. They reasoned that because of increased functional demands and stresses on the surrounding joints after an arthrodesis there is an increase in abnormal motion and chronic loading of these joints, which lead to the development of osteoarthritis. The joints involved in their series included subtalar joint (Fig. 6), talonavicular joint, tarsometatarsal joint, naviculocuneiform, calcaneocuboid, and first metatarsophalangeal joint, in decreasing order of prevalence. Although they found correlation between foot function and the grade of the degenerative changes on the radiographs, they could not correlate pain and grade of arthritis. Arguably, ankle arthrodesis still stands as a standard treatment, with a caveat that foot function does deteriorate with time. Deterioration in function along with increasing pain is often difficult to deal with by bracing alone. One surgical option involves fusion of the adjacent joints, however. The results of such pantalar fusions are often guarded and fraught with complications [49,55].

Leg length inequalities

Limb length is often compromised during an attempted ankle arthrodesis to achieve a solid union. Postoperatively, limb muscle atrophy occurs as a result of long periods of immobilization. Limb shortening and limb atrophy are expected outcomes at the end of a successful ankle arthrodesis. Several studies have shown that leg length inequalities up to 2.5 cm or 1 inch are

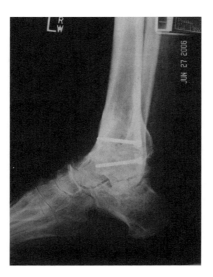

Fig. 6. Lateral radiograph demonstrates subtalar arthritis 8 years after an arthrodesis of the ankle.

often well tolerated by patients through the use of shoe lifts [56,57]. If the limb length inequality happens to be more than 3 cm, however, then a surgical option is the treatment of choice. In their article on treatment of malunions and nonunions after an ankle fusion, Katsenis and colleagues [24] showed that this could be done effectively with the help of a circular fine wire frame with good predictable results. They described this technique using distraction osteogenesis proximally closer to the knee (with a revision ankle arthrodesis at the distal end if an associated nonunion or malunion is present). With the help of the circular frame, it is often possible not only to achieve limb length correction but also to correct any three-dimensional or multiplanar problems at the ankle simultaneously.

Ankle arthroplasty: a salvage option

In patients with painful ankle arthrodesis with or without a nonunion, in the absence of infection, an ankle arthroplasty is a possible salvage option. It is reserved for patients with adequate bone stock remaining to support an arthroplasty and allow for adequate ingrowth fixation, especially patients with associated degenerative changes in the subtalar joints who would otherwise require a pantalar arthrodesis, which requires oxygen consumption for gait akin to a patient with a below-the-knee or transtibial amputation [49,55]. In their series of 23 patients who had undergone such a conversion from fusion to total ankle arthroplasty, Greisberg and colleagues [29] reported overall higher satisfaction scores in all the patients after conversion to a total ankle arthroplasty. They did demonstrate higher American Orthopaedic Foot and Ankle Society hindfoot scores for the group converted because of associated subtalar arthritis than those done for a painful fusion. Similarly, Barg and Hintermann [58] recently reported conversion for 29 painful ankle arthrodeses (27 for pain, 2 for nonunion) to ankle arthroplasty using a three-component system with high patient satisfaction regarding pain relief and regained function.

Summary

With evolved techniques and methods of fixation, ankle fusion has become a successful surgery with high fusion rates and predictably high satisfaction rates. As a result, arthrodesis of the ankle remains the gold standard for surgical management of end-stage ankle arthritis. Complications and failures do occur for various reasons, however, as reviewed in the article. They often can be avoided or reduced with proper surgical planning and technique. Proper patient selection becomes key to successful surgery. The surgical techniques involved in the primary fusion and the salvage options are technically challenging and should be undertaken by orthopedic surgeons well trained within the foot and ankle subspecialty. A surgeon performing a revision arthrodesis also must be well versed in all salvage options, with an in-depth understanding of the mechanics, alignment, and function of the ankle foot complex. A well thought out approach to the failed ankle arthrodesis can result in return to function and successful outcomes. A below-the-knee amputation remains the final salvage for the recurrently failed ankle arthrodesis.

References

[1] Albert E. Zur resektion des kniegelenkes. Weiner Medizinische Press 1879;20:705–8, [In German].
[2] Ahlberg A, Henricson AS. Late results of ankle fusion. Acta Orthop Scand 1981;52:103–5.
[3] Mazur JM, Schwartz E, Simon SR. Ankle arthrodesis: long-term follow-up with gait analysis. J Bone Joint Surg Am 1979;61:964–75.
[4] Boobbyer GN. The long-term results of ankle arthrodesis. Acta Orthop Scand 1981;52:107–10.
[5] Lynch AF, Bourne RB, Rorabeck CH. The long-term results of ankle arthrodesis. J Bone Joint Surg Br 1988;70:113–6.
[6] Coester LM, Saltzman CL, Leupold J, et al. Long-term results following ankle arthrodesis for post-traumatic arthritis. J Bone Joint Surg Am 2001;83-A(2):219–28.
[7] Muir DC, Amendola A, Saltzman CL. Long-term outcome of ankle arthrodesis. Foot Ankle Clin 2002;7(4):703–8.
[8] Thomas R, Daniels TR, Parker K. Gait analysis and functional outcomes following ankle arthrodesis for isolated ankle arthritis. J Bone Joint Surg Am 2006;88(3):526–35.
[9] Saltzman CL. Perspective on total ankle replacement. Foot Ankle Clin 2000;5(4):761–75.
[10] Neufeld SK, Lee TH. Total ankle arthroplasty: indications, results, and biomechanical rationale. Am J Orthop 2000;29(8):593–602.
[11] Kile TA, Donnelly RE, Gehrke JC, et al. Tibiotalocalcaneal arthrodesis with an intramedullaary device. Foot Ankle Int 1994;15(12):669–73.
[12] Papa J, Myerson M, Girard P. Salvage, with arthrodesis, in intractable diabetic neuropathic arthropathy of the foot and ankle. J Bone Joint Surg Am 1993;75(7):1056–66.
[13] Pinzur MS, Kelikian A. Charcot ankle fusion with a retrograde locked intramedullary nail. Foot Ankle Int 1997;18(11):699–704.
[14] Morgan CD, Henke JA, Bailey RW, et al. Long-term results of tibiotalar arthrodesis. J Bone Joint Surg Am 1985;67:546–50.
[15] Fuchs S, Sandmann C, Skawara A, et al. Quality of life 20 years after arthrodesis of the ankle: a study of adjacent joints. J Bone Joint Surg Br 2003;85(7):994–8.
[16] Salem KH, Kinz L, Schmelz A. Ankle arthrodesis using Ilizarov ring fixators: a review of 22 cases. Foot Ankle Int 2006;27(10):764–70.
[17] Thomas R, Daniels TR. Ankle arthritis. J Bone Joint Surg Am 2003;85-A(5):923–36.
[18] Said E, Hunka L, Siller TN. Where ankle fusion stands today. J Bone Joint Surg Br 1978;60-B(2):211–4.
[19] Lance EM, Paval A, Fries I, et al. Arthrodesis of the ankle joint: a follow-up study. Clin Orthop Relat Res 1979;(142):146–58.
[20] Kenzora JE, Simmons SC, Burgess AR, et al. External fixation arthrodesis of the ankle joint following trauma. Foot Ankle 1986;7(1):49–61.
[21] Morrey BF, Wiedeman GP. Complications and long-term results of ankle arthrodeses following trauma. J Bone Joint Surg Am 1980;62(5):777–84.
[22] Ratliff AH. Compression arthrodesis of the ankle. J Bone Joint Surg Br 1959;41-B:524–34.
[23] Scranton PE, Fu FH, Brown TD. Ankle arthrodesis: a comparative clinical and biomechanical evaluation. Clin Orthop Relat Res 1980;(151):234–43.
[24] Katsenis D, Bhave A, Paley D. Treatment of malunion and nonunion at the site of an ankle fusion with the Ilizarov apparatus. J Bone Joint Surg Am 2005;87(2):302–9.

[25] Mendonca DA, Cosker T, Makwana NK. Vacuum-assisted closure to aid wound healing in foot and ankle surgery. Foot Ankle Int 2005;26(9):761–6.

[26] Hagen RJ. Ankle arthrodesis: problems and pitfalls. Clin Orthop Relat Res 1986;(202): 152–62.

[27] Buck P, Morrey BF, Chao EY. The optimum position of arthrodesis of the ankle: a gait study of the knee and ankle. J Bone Joint Surg Am 1987;69(7):1052–62.

[28] King HA, Watkins TB, Samuelson KM. Analysis of foot position in ankle arthrodesis and its influence on gait. Foot Ankle 1980;1(1):44–9.

[29] Greisberg J, Assal M, Flueckiger G, et al. Takedown of ankle fusion and conversion to total ankle replacement. Clin Orthop Relat Res 2004;(424):80–8.

[30] Haddad SL, Coetzee JC, Estok R, et al. Intermediate and long-term outcomes of total ankle arthroplasty and ankle arthrodesis: a systematic review of the literature. J Bone Joint Surg Am 2007;89(9):1899–905.

[31] Scranton PE. Use of internal compression in arthrodesis of the ankle. J Bone Joint Surg Am 1985;67(4):550–5.

[32] Stewart MJ, Beeler TC, McConnell JC. Compression arthrodesis of the ankle: evaluation of a cosmetic modification. J Bone Joint Surg Am 1983;65(2):219–25.

[33] Hallock H. Arthrodesis of the ankle joint for old painful fractures. J Bone Joint Surg Am 1945;27:49–58.

[34] Monroe MT, Beals TC, Manoli A. Clinical outcome of arthrodesis of the ankle using rigid internal fixation with cancellous screws. Foot Ankle Int 1999;20(4):227–31.

[35] Sowa DT, Krackow KA. Ankle fusion: a new technique of internal fixation using a compression blade plate. Foot Ankle 1989;9(5):232–40.

[36] Cierny G, Cook WG, Mader JT. Ankle arthrodesis in the presence of ongoing sepsis: indications, methods, and results. Orthop Clin North Am 1989;20(4):709–21.

[37] Hayes JT, Gross HP, Dow S. Surgery for paralytic defects secondary to myelomeningocele and myelodysplasia. J Bone Joint Surg Am 1964;46:1577–97.

[38] Frey C, Halikus NM, Vu-Rose T, et al. A review of ankle arthrodesis: predisposing factors to nonunion. Foot Ankle Int 1994;15(11):581–4.

[39] Anderson JG, Coetzee JC, Hansen ST. Revision ankle fusion using internal compression arthrodesis with screw fixation. Foot Ankle Int 1997;18(5):300–9.

[40] Cobb TK, Gabrielsen TA, Campbell DC, et al. Cigarette smoking and nonunion after ankle arthrodesis. Foot Ankle Int 1994;15(2):64–7.

[41] Haverstock BD, Mandracchia VJ. Cigarette smoking and bone healing: implications in foot and ankle surgery. J Foot Ankle Surg 1998;37(1):69–74.

[42] Kitaoka HB, Anderson PJ, Morrey BF. Revision of ankle arthrodesis with external fixation for non-union. J Bone Joint Surg Am 1992;74(8):1191–200.

[43] Perlman MH, Thordarson DB. Ankle fusion in a high risk population: an assessment of non-union risk factors. Foot Ankle Int 1999;20(8):491–6.

[44] Pinzur MS. Current concepts review: Charcot arthropathy of the foot and ankle. Foot Ankle Int 2007;28(8):952–9.

[45] Bibbo C, Goldberg JW. Infectious and healing complications after elective orthopaedic foot and ankle surgery during tumor necrosis factor-alpha inhibition therapy. Foot Ankle Int 2004;25(5):331–5.

[46] Saltzman C, Lightfoot A, Amendola A. PEMF as treatment for delayed healing of foot and ankle arthrodesis. Foot Ankle Int 2004;25(11):771–3.

[47] Perry CR, Pearson RL, Miller GA. Accuracy of cultures of material from swabbing of the superficial aspect of the wound and needle biopsy in the preoperative assessment of osteomyelitis. J Bone Joint Surg Am 1991;73(5):745–9.

[48] Saltzman CL. Salvage of diffuse ankle osteomyelitis by single-stage resection and circumferential frame compression arthrodesis. Iowa Orthop J 2005;25:47–52.

[49] Acosta R, Ushiba J, Cracchiolo A. The results of a primary and staged pantalar arthrodesis and tibiotalocalcaneal arthrodesis in adult patients. Foot Ankle Int 2000;21(3):182–94.

[50] Richter D, Hahn MP, Laun RA, et al. Arthrodesis of the infected ankle and subtalar joint: technique, indications, and results of 45 consecutive cases. J Trauma 1999;47(6):1072–8.

[51] Thordarson DB, Patzakis MJ, Holtom P, et al. Salvage of the septic ankle with concomitant tibial osteomyelitis. Foot Ankle Int 1997;18(3):151–6.

[52] Kollig E, Esenwein SA, Muhr G, et al. Fusion of the septic ankle: experience with 15 cases using hybrid external fixation. J Trauma 2003;55(4):685–91.

[53] Kitaoka HB, Patzer GL. Arthrodesis for the treatment of arthrosis of the ankle and osteonecrosis of the talus. J Bone Joint Surg Am 1998;80(3):370–9.

[54] Boer R, Mader K, Pennig D, et al. Tibiotalocalcaneal arthrodesis using a reamed retrograde locking nail. Clin Orthop Relat Res 2007;463:151–6.

[55] Papa JA, Myerson MS. Pantalar and tibiotalocalcaneal arthrodesis for post-traumatic osteoarthrosis of the ankle and hindfoot. J Bone Joint Surg Am 1992;74(7):1042–9.

[56] Gross RH. Leg length discrepancy: how much is too much? Orthopedics 1978;1(4):307–10.

[57] Moseley CF. Leg-length discrepancy. In: Morrissy RT, Weinstein SL, editors. Lovell & Winter's pediatric orthopaedics. vol. 2. 6th edition. Philadelphia: Lippincott Williams & Wilkins; 2006. p. 1234–6.

[58] Barg AJ, Hintermann B. Take down of painful ankle fusion and conversion into total ankle arthroplasty. Presented at the AAOS 75th Annual meeting. San Francisco, 2008.

ELSEVIER
SAUNDERS

Foot Ankle Clin N Am
13 (2008) 417–442

FOOT AND
ANKLE CLINICS

Management of the Varus Arthritic Ankle

Michael S. Hennessy, BSc, FRCSEd (Tr&Orth)[a],*,
Andrew P. Molloy, FRCS (Tr&Orth)[b],
Edward V. Wood, FRCS (Tr&Orth)[a]

[a]*Department of Orthopaedics, Wirral University Hospitals NHS Trust, Upton,
Wirral CH49 5PE, United Kingdom*
[b]*Department of Orthopaedics, University Hospital Aintree,
Liverpool L9 7AL, United Kingdom*

Deformity in the coronal plane is a common feature of the arthritic ankle. Varus malalignment tends to result from chronic lateral ligamentous insufficiency (whether recognized and symptomatic or subclinical), but such deformity also can be seen in inflammatory joint disease, affecting 15% of subjects in one study [1]. Frequently the hindfoot and forefoot are in varus also.

To achieve lasting success, correction of these associated deformities is an essential part of whatever treatment modality is considered appropriate for the arthritic ankle of an individual patient. This article attempts to give an overview of the techniques that have been and are currently used. The authors have tried to be nonprescriptive, because the specific cause and presentation as well as the experience and skills of the treating surgeon influence the treatment of each patient. The authors believe that the varus arthritic ankle deformity can present some of the most challenging problems in foot and ankle surgery. The goal of intervention always is to create a pain-free, plantigrade, shoeable foot.

Anatomy

The specific anatomy and biomechanics of the ankle joint present unique problems and technical difficulties. Unlike the hip and knee joint, several other joints are in close proximity to the ankle joint, and their movements

---

* Corresponding author.
E-mail address: mchenno@btinternet.com (M.S. Hennessy).

1083-7515/08/$ - see front matter © 2008 Elsevier Inc. All rights reserved.
doi:10.1016/j.fcl.2008.04.006

are coupled to those of the ankle joint. Deformity and abnormalities in these joints therefore have a direct affect on the ankle joint. The association of sagittal-plane movement with axial rotation both within and without the ankle create unique couplings of motion that make ankle arthroplasty inherently more challenging than arthroplasty of the hip and knee. The normal ankle joint possesses a large (tibiotalar) contact area that is inherently stable under static load. Passive ankle stability under weight-bearing conditions depends substantially on the articular surface geometry, and geometric abnormality affects joint kinematics during locomotion [2]. Dynamic stability, however, depends on the integrity and normal functioning of the supporting ligaments and musculotendinous units crossing the joint or those adjacent to it. The relative rarity of primary degenerative disease of the ankle attests to the ankle's inherent mechanical efficiency. Minor trauma or subtle changes in alignment can result in articular degeneration, however.

Assessment and preoperative considerations

Assessment of the varus ankle begins, as always, with assessment of gait and the lower limbs as a whole, but particular attention is given to the relationship of the ankle to the foot. Deformity in the coronal plane is compensated by the subtalar joint; deformity in the sagittal plane is compensated in the ankle. When the deformity becomes chronic, the compensatory movement that attempts to maintain a plantigrade foot also may become permanent. It is important to recognize these adaptive changes in the foot. The etiology of a cavovarus deformity is multifactorial, from subtle deformity, thought to be idiopathic, to recognized neurologic conditions, such as hereditary motor sensory neuropathy. The recognition of an associated deformity in the foot or leg is vital to the successful treatment of the varus ankle. The more common considerations are

- The condition of contralateral limb (eg, for rehabilitation)
- The condition of ipsilateral hindfoot (Are additional procedures needed?)
- Plantarflexed first ray
- Heel varus
- Forefoot pronation with or without clawing of the lesser toes
- Tight tendo Achilles/gastrocnemius complex

Some or all of these problems may need to be taken into account and corrected in addition to the ankle deformity, either at the time of the index ankle procedure or separately.

Causes of the varus arthritic ankle

Box 1 outlines the causes of the varus arthritic ankle.

Box 1. Causes of the varus arthritic ankle

Posttraumatic
- Malunion of tibial shaft fracture
- After pilon fracture
- Complications of talar fracture (eg, Avascular Necrosis (AVN)), calcaneal fractures, transverse tarsal or midfoot (Lisfranc) fracture/dislocations
- Compartment syndromes
- Lateral ligament insufficiency

Degenerative
- Varus knee arthritis
- Rheumatoid arthritis

Neurologic
- Hereditary motor sensory neuropathy
- Stroke/cerebrovascular accident
- Central and peripheral nerve disorders
- Polio
- Congenital talipes equinovarus

Arthrodesis, arthroplasty, or joint-sparing techniques?

Once nonoperative measures have been exhausted, the surgical options are joint-sparing techniques, arthrodesis, and arthroplasty. The arguments for and against each technique and considerations to be borne in mind are outlined in the following sections.

Joint-sparing techniques

Supramalleolar osteotomy
The relationship between varus deformity of the ankle, subsequent changes in joint biomechanics, and their association with osteoarthritis (OA) have been covered extensively in a number of recent review articles [3–6], but few clinical series have reported the results of this technique [7–12].

Correction of the deformity in varus OA ankles improves function and symptoms, in selected patient groups, and thus delays or obviates the need for either total ankle replacement (TAR) or arthrodesis. Normalizing or slight overcorrection of the joint orientation allows unloading of the damaged or abnormal cartilage and transfer of the load to the remaining, healthy, cartilage.

The indications for correction have yet to be well defined because of limited clinical experience. In general, symptomatic, degenerative joint disease with a deviation of more than 10° from normal in the coronal plane and preservation of the lateral articular cartilage should be corrected. Pagenstert and colleagues [10], however, offer an algorithm for decision making in medial and lateral ankle OA.

Multiple methods of correcting a varus ankle have been described, using either a medial opening wedge or a lateral closing wedge osteotomy. The former technique is the default technique in most current series. The resultant defect requires bone grafting and stabilization, usually with a plate, although Kirschner wires, intramedullary nails, external fixators, and circular frames are all options (Figs. 1 and 2).

Takakura's group [7–9] has published three articles reporting the results of supramalleolar osteotomy. The first, in 1995, presented the results of a low tibial osteotomy for varus OA in 18 ankles, with 3 having concurrent lateral ligament reconstruction [7]. The mean age of patients was 59 years. The mean follow-up of 6 years, 11 months revealed excellent results in 6 patients, good results in 9 patients, fair results in 3 patients, and no poor results. A further article in 1998 reported nine patients who underwent an opening wedge osteotomy for posttraumatic varus deformity of the ankle [8]. The mean follow-up was 7 years, 4 months, with excellent results in four patients, good results in two patients, and fair results in three patients. This series included four children under the age of 16 years; the mean age of the five adults was 51 years. Most recently Tanaka and colleagues [9] reported 19 good or excellent results in a series of 26 medial opening wedge osteotomies. The best results were in patients who had early or limited OA, with some showing signs of recovery of the medial joint space.

Pagenstert and colleagues [10] reported a series of 35 patients who had posttraumatic OA with varus or valgus deformities. Varus ankles underwent

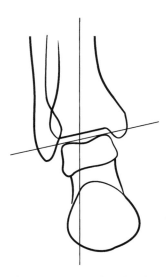

Fig. 1. A varus ankle deformity.

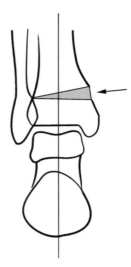

Fig. 2. Varus deformity corrected by an opening wedge osteotomy.

correction with an opening wedge osteotomy, bone graft, and plate stabilization. They reported reduced pain and a significantly improved range of motion in the varus ankle. There was a 29% revision rate, with 9% conversion to TAR at less than 2 years.

Similar results have also been reported by Cheng and colleagues [11] and Stamatis and colleagues [12], with both reporting functional improvement after correction of deformity.

Supramalleolar osteotomy probably is an underutilized technique, because the evidence cited previously shows that it can slow or halt the symptomatic progression of OA, without preventing future surgery, should it become necessary. The described series are small, however, and surgeons are likely to be cautious until further large-scale series are available.

Hindfoot osteotomy

The use of hindfoot osteotomy for the correction of varus ankle OA is not well reported in the literature. Lateral ligament instability and hindfoot varus often are associated and can lead to varus OA. They may be the result of an underlying cavus foot deformity, which must be looked for in the initial assessment, as outlined previously.

The aim of hindfoot osteotomy is to move the weight-bearing axis so that the ankle no longer tips into varus. Doing so involves the use of a lateral displacement calcaneal osteotomy, which may require augmentation with a lateral ligament repair or reconstruction. If the varus is driven by the forefoot, a dorsiflexion osteotomy of the first ray or dorsiflexion tarsometatarsal joint arthrodesis is undertaken.

Arthrodesis

Arthrodesis certainly is the most established technique in the treatment of end-stage ankle arthritis, the goals being pain relief, deformity correction, and maintenance of hindfoot stability.

Gait analysis and clinical studies have shown the preferred position of ankle fusion to be plantigrade, with 5° of hindfoot valgus, external rotation of 5° to 10° or comparable with that of the contralateral extremity, and the talus translated posteriorly in relation to the tibia to reduce the lever arm [13,14]. With a well-positioned arthrodesis, gait efficiency achieves 90% of normal, and the energy expenditure required is only 3% greater than for a normal counterpart at a similar pace of walking [15].

The mild valgus positioning of the hindfoot allows pronation of the foot, thus unlocking the mid-tarsal joints, which are used as a compensatory mechanism, allowing more natural motion of the hindfoot [16–18]. This result was demonstrated clinically by Morgan and colleagues [19], who showed increased mid-tarsal motion after ankle arthrodesis. Buck and colleagues [20] also found that fusion in a slight valgus position permitted markedly more varus–valgus motion of the hindfoot than possible with fusion in a varus position. Arthrodesis in a varus position has a detrimental effect, because a supinated, locked hindfoot with lateral column overload will result. Helm [21] demonstrated significantly inferior Mazur scores in ankles fused in varus or valgus, in comparison with those fused in a neutral position (67.4 versus 73.9, respectively). Varus positioning also has been shown to be a risk factor for non-union after arthrodesis [22].

Arthrodesis techniques

A multitude of different ankle arthrodesis techniques have been described, including Dowel arthrodesis [23], inlay grafts [24], onlay grafts [25,26], staples [27], screw fixation [28–31], T-plates [32], angle blade plates [33–35], intramedullary nails [36–38], and external fixation [39,40]—and this list is far from exhaustive! More recently, limited open and arthroscopic techniques have been published [24,41–47].

Open techniques specific to the varus ankle

Smith and Wood [48] reported on 25 ankle arthrodeses in patients who had OA and a coronal-plane deformity greater than 20°, 20 of whom had a varus deformity. Open arthrodesis via an anterior approach was undertaken, with two 6.5-mm parallel, cannulated screws providing compressive internal fixation. A transarticular resection osteotomy of the fibula was required in 13 of these patients. A further four patients required a proximal dorsal wedge osteotomy of the first metatarsal for fixed plantarflexion deformity associated with the varus. They report good results with this technique: there was 1 non-union (4%), and correction within 5° of neutral was achieved 18 in of the 25 patients (mean correction, 25°), along with improvement in the American Orthopaedics Foot and Ankle Society (AOFAS) scores (a postoperative pain score of 10.5, versus 35.2 preoperatively, and a postoperative function score of 43.7, versus 25.5 preoperatively).

In another series, Fortin and colleagues [49] reported on 10 patients who had cavovarus feet with lateral ankle ligament instability and varying degrees of OA. Of these, six patients (eight cavovarus feet) who had end-stage OA in varus ankles underwent arthrodesis. Three also required a dorsiflexion osteotomy of the first metatarsal because of a persistently plantar flexed first ray. They achieved good results with neutral or slight valgus heel alignment in all but one patient and an improvement in functional scores in all patients.

Arthroscopic techniques

Arthroscopic ankle arthrodesis (AAA) has become more popular as surgeons have gained experience in ankle arthroscopy, and a standard technique is well described, with few significant variations, by several authors [42,43,46,50–52].

AAA has proven advantages over open techniques: although the rates of fusion between open and arthroscopic techniques are comparable, arthroscopic surgery results in less blood loss, lower morbidity, shorter hospital stay, and more rapid mobilization [52]. Myerson and Quill [51] also demonstrated a faster time to union, with a mean time of 8.7 weeks in the arthroscopic group and 14.5 weeks in the open group. Most authors, however, recommend that the use of AAA be restricted to ankles with little or no coronal plane deformity ($<10°$–$15°$), because obtaining a significant correction is more difficult arthroscopically, and an in situ fusion usually is performed [42,43,45,51,53].

Arthroscopic techniques specific to the varus ankle

Others have addressed more significant deformity using arthroscopic methods with encouraging results.

Cannon and colleagues [31], in 2004, reported results of AAA comparing immediate and restricted postoperative weight bearing. They showed a 100% union rate at 4 months in both groups. Although their article did not concentrate specifically on AAA with coronal plane deformity, it is clear that significant deformity was addressed, with a maximum varus deformity of 27° in their series. Their surgical technique for deformity correction was not covered in depth, but their practice was to perform an examination under anesthetic with fluoroscopic control; if the talus could be corrected to neutral with traction, an AAA could be undertaken.

In 2005, Winson and colleagues [54] reported a series of 105 AAAs in patients who had coronal-plane deformity ranging from 22° valgus to 28° varus. A standard arthroscopic technique was used with fixation using parallel, 6.5-mm, cannulated screws from the medial side. If the heel still remained in excessive varus or valgus, this deviation was corrected with an os-calcis osteotomy. This procedure was done in four cases. They obtained good to excellent results in 83 patients, with a non-union rate of 7.6%. They concluded that the indications for AAA can be extended to include patients who have deformity once experience has been gained with minimally deformed ankles. They also recommend that, when an uncorrectable pronation or supination deformity of the forefoot is found during assessment, an open arthrodesis be undertaken that then may be extended into other joints.

More recently, Gougoulias and colleagues [55] reported a retrospective study comparing 78 AAAs in two groups. Group A contained 48 patients who had minor coronal-plane deformity (<15°; mean, 5.6°). Group B contained 30 patients who had a major deformity (>15° and up to 45°; mean, 24.7°). In both groups resection of the articular surfaces was performed in the standard fashion. In group B, further debridement of the tibial surface was performed to correct the deformity. Fixation was with two or three parallel, 6.5-mm, cannulated screws. Four patients in group B required concomitant subtalar arthrodesis. There was no significant difference between the two groups: there was one non-union in each group, and good alignment was achieved with a mean of 0.7° valgus in group A and of 0.4° valgus in group B. The authors conclude that AAA is appropriate and advocate its use in patients who have OA with a marked deformity.

Although increasingly large deformities can be addressed arthroscopically, with good results, it is clear that this approach should be undertaken only by those with large experience in AAA. In the author's opinion, the default technique for fusion in arthritic ankles with a large varus deformity remains an open arthrodesis. In most surgeons' hands an AAA can be used to achieve an in situ fusion with debridement of the joint surfaces and a limited capacity for correction. Open techniques readily allow a more radical correction of the deformity, either through resection of the tibia/talar surfaces or with additional techniques such as a fibula resection osteotomy.

Outcomes

Union rates from ankle arthrodesis in the literature range from 60% to 100% [28,39,56]. With modern internal and external fixation techniques, the best recent results have been reported as ranging from 95% to 100% [19,23,29,32,35,36,42,43,45,46,48,51]. Although, other than the few studies mentioned previously (Smith and Wood [48], Fortin and colleagues [49]), most reports do not address the specifics of varus ankle arthrodesis directly, it is recognized that successful rates of arthrodesis are diminished in subgroups of patients who have comorbidities. Smoking, for example, has been reported to be associated with a further 16-fold increase in non-union rates [57].

Historical articles on the outcome of ankle arthrodesis considered a successful outcome to be union of the fusion. With evolution of modern scoring systems, such as the AOFAS hindfoot and ankle scoring system in 1994 [58], more emphasis has been placed on the patient's subjective analysis of the functional outcome.

Arthroplasty

There are no statistically powerful randomized trials directly comparing the functional results or the complication rates of ankle arthrodesis versus total ankle arthroplasty. The meta-analysis of intermediate and long-term results of these modes of treatments by Haddad and colleagues [59] gave AOFAS ankle hindfoot scores of 78.2 (95% confidence interval, 71.9–84.5) for arthroplasty and 75.6% for ankle arthrodesis (95% confidence interval, 71.6–79.9).

Functional analysis

After ankle arthrodesis, gait historically has been reported as relatively normal, especially with the use of orthotics such as a negative heel, a declination angle sole, and a solid ankle cushion heel [18,60]. Ankle arthrodesis does change the efficiency of gait in walking barefoot, however. Waters and colleagues [15] demonstrated only a 3% increase in oxygen consumption in patients who had undergone ankle arthrodesis but a 10% overall decrease in efficiency of gait and a 16% decrease in gait velocity. Gait velocity is affected by the foreshortened strides secondary to loss of sagittal-plane motion. Preventing this result has been one of the main objectives of inventors of total ankle arthroplasty prostheses. The ankle does not move as a simple hinge joint but rather moves as a complex hinge coupled with three-dimensional motions: plantar flexion and dorsiflexion are coupled with valgus, varus, external rotation, and internal rotation [61]. Ankle arthroplasty cannot hope to recreate these vectors of motion, but the biomechanics that it does provide are closer to normal motion than obtained with an ankle arthrodesis. An in vitro study by Michelson and colleagues [61] showed that, although coupled motions are not significantly different from those in normal ankle controls, there was increased hysteresis in both the axial and coronal planes. It thus was hypothesized that subtle changes may promote abnormal stress transfers at the ankle, promoting early implant failure. Ranges of motion achieved by patients who have undergone ankle arthroplasty range from 17° to 28° in the literature, and these ranges are little different from preoperative values [62–65]. In normal gait, an ankle range of motion of 14° is required for the stance phase of gait, although a range of motion of 37° to 56° is required for normal ability to ascend and descend stairs. Therefore, if the published mean ranges of motion are achieved, patients should be able to return to daily activities without the use of orthotics, providing these activities do not involve frequent or abnormal stair use. Despite these range-of-motion results, Doets and colleagues [66] reported that gait velocity was reduced by 6% in patients who had undergone ankle arthroplasty as compared with normal controls. Also although the kinematics in the joints throughout the leg was nearly normal, ground reaction forces and electromyographic activity did not normalize fully. An improvement, but not normalization, of electromyographic activity also was reported, by Valderrabano and colleagues [67]. They also demonstrated statistically significant improvement in plantar flexion and dorsiflexion torque, as compared with the preoperative state, in patients who had undergone arthroplasty.

Outcomes

The decrease in sagittal-plane motion in patients who have undergone ankle arthrodesis is reported to average 60% to 70% [68,69]. This loss of motion is compensated primarily by an increase in transverse tarsal and midfoot movement. Sealey and colleagues [70] showed prospectively a mean increase of 4° in midfoot range of motion and of 5.5° in subtalar movement after a mean follow-up of 2.2 years. They also showed impingement of the posterior part of the posterior facet of the subtalar joint, which may account for the well-reported incidence of hindfoot OA [56,71,72]. Koefed and Sturup [73] reported subtalar osteoarthritis in 5 of 14 patients who had undergone ankle arthrodesis at 7 years follow-up and no evidence of subtalar arthritis in the 14 patients who underwent arthroplasty. The meta-analysis by SooHoo and colleagues [74] reported that the rate of subtalar arthritis at 5 years is 2.8% in patients who had undergone an ankle arthrodesis but was only 0.7% in those who had undergone ankle arthroplasty. Progression to a pantalar arthrodesis obviously causes a much larger functional deficit and probably leads to dissatisfaction in patients. Although, Greisberg and colleagues [75] showed good results in taking down an arthrodesis and conversion to arthroplasty, these results have not been reproduced on a widespread basis and would not be considered standard treatment. Survival rates of modern ankle prostheses have improved dramatically since total ankle arthroplasty was performed by Lord and Marrotte [76] in 1970. Five-year survival rates range from 70% to 98% for mobile-bearing designs and from 80% to 97% for fixed-bearing designs [62–64,77–83]. Most long-term prosthesis survival rates exceeding 10 years have been reported by the inventors of the respective prostheses. These include 92% survival at 12 years for the Buechel-Pappas prosthesis (Endotec, South Orange, New Jersey), 95% 12-year survival for the Scandinavian Total Ankle Replacement (STAR) prosthesis (Waldemar Link GmbH & Co., Hamburg, Germany), and 85% survival at 10 years for the Agility prosthesis (DePuy, Warsaw, Indiana) [63,78,80]. Wood and Deakin [65], however, also reported an 83% overall survival rate at 10 years for a cohort of Buechel-Pappas and STAR prostheses. Of great interest are the recent reports and results from National Joint Registries. Henricson and colleagues [84] reported a 98% survival at 5 years from the Swedish Joint Registry. Hosman and colleagues [85] reported a 7% revision rate at a mean of 28 months with a cumulative 5-year survivorship of 85% from the New Zealand Registry. Fevang and colleagues [86] reported an overall 5-year survival rate of 89% and a 10-year survival rate of 76%. These three Joint Registry results provide excellent clinical governance standards for the survival rates that should be obtained from total ankle arthroplasty.

Arthroplasty and varus deformity

Few authors have correlated initial coronal-plane deformity with long-term outcome. Doets and colleagues [1] reported 90% survivorship at 8 years in neutrally aligned ankles versus 48% in ankles with deformity greater than 10°. Wood and colleagues [87] reported an overall survivorship of 88% in rheumatoid patients. If only patients who had well-preserved alignment were considered, however, the 10-year survivorship in this study was 97%. In another study of 200 STAR prostheses by Wood and colleagues [65], a far higher incidence of polyethylene edge loading was found in the presence of deformity. This finding led to the recommendation that deformity greater than 15° be considered a relative contraindication to ankle arthroplasty. More recent studies have shown good short-term results in patients who have a preoperative coronal-plane deformity greater than 10°. Hobson and Dhar [88] showed no significant difference in the survivorship in patients grouped into coronal-plane deformities of more or less than 10° at a mean of 3 years using a variety of realignment techniques. These results correlate with the results from single-method (ie, medial malleolar osteotomy or deltoid release) reports [1,77,89]. Preoperative assessment of the varus ankle is critical for performing a successful ankle arthroplasty. If a plantigrade foot with a neutrally aligned ankle is not achieved, early failure is likely to occur. In severe cases, talar tilting will occur. Talar tilting produces large stresses on the polyethylene bearing system, leading to increased generation of wear particles and even fracture of the polyethylene. In severe cases, especially in the presence of osteopenia, subsidence of the either the tibia or the talar implant may occur. Even if obvious radiographic talar tilting does not occur with the residual varus, forces will be concentrated on the medial side of the polyethylene liner. The large shearing axial forces across the ankle will exceed the mechanical strength of the polyethylene, thereby propagating wear. Studies have shown that compressive forces across the ankle during normal gait exceed five times the body weight [90,91]. Arthritic varus deformity of the ankle often presents with narrowing of the medial joint space and bony erosion (normally from the tibia) with typical sloping of the medial malleolus or with a relatively normal medial joint space with lateral opening caused by gross lateral ligament instability. Usually, however, the patient has a combination of the two problems.

One always should be mindful of the possibility that lateral ligament insufficiency is being masked by the stiffness of the arthrosis, if there is any lateral opening. This is particularly true if there is a large anterior cheilus, which can prevent any anterior subluxation. Once the cheilus is removed during the initial approach to the arthroplasty, lateral ligamentous integrity should be reassessed. A variety of methods have been proposed for the treatment of the varus ankle when performing an arthroplasty. The simplest scenario is of mild medial bony erosion with an intact lateral ligament complex. In these cases a planar distal tibial bony cut just proximal to the medial defect should correct the deformity. This correction necessitates a deeper polyethylene insert, and the correction obviously is easier with a prosthesis that has the sufficient range of modularity. Using this technique in this type of varus deformity usually negates the need for significant soft tissue balancing. Caution should be exercised in larger defects, however, especially with lateral ligament insufficiency. With these deficiencies excess bone resection is unlikely to correct the deformity fully. Further resection of the bone stock will complicate revision arthroplasty or arthrodesis if the primary prosthesis fails. In fact, this additional resection can lead to an increased rate of failure because of subsidence of the tibial component. Resection of the subchondral plate alone reduces compressive resistance of bone by 30%–50%. Additional resection will further weaken it, with a 1 cm resection producing a 70%–90% reduction in compressive resistance.

A variety of methods have been described for the correction of varus deformity secondary to lateral ligament insufficiency. Doets and colleagues [1] described a lengthening medial malleolar osteotomy in 15 arthroplasties (Fig. 3). At a mean follow-up of 5 years, the mean AOFAS score increased from 30.8 to 81.0. There was revision of one of the prostheses, and there were six reoperations in four of the patients (two triple arthrodeses, one Dwyer osteotomy, one supramalleolar osteotomy, two arthroscopic

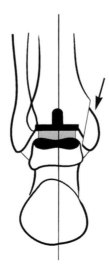

Fig. 3. Medial malleolar osteotomy.

debridements, and one open debridement). Kofoed [92] described a talar sculpting resection with a lateral ligament reconstruction if necessary. Several authors have proposed various methods of deltoid release, with or without lateral reconstruction. It also has been noted that, especially when using the Agility prosthesis, medial positioning of the talar component lateralizes the ground reaction and can compensate for a mild residual varus [93].

The authors of this article prefer combination of bony and soft tissue procedures. The ankle joint is distracted using leverage from a broad osteotome after the initial approach using toothed laminar spreaders in the medial side of the joint after the distal tibia cut. This distraction may stretch out any mild contraction of the medial structures. Further compensation for medial erosion is achieved using distal tibia cut. They have found the intramedullary realignment jig of the Mobility prosthesis (DePuy, Leeds, United Kingdom) useful in providing an accurate cut perpendicular to the mechanical axis of the tibia. Often this cut balances the ankle into a plantargrade position, even if there was some relative lateral laxity before this cut. If the joint space is still trapezoidal after resection, a segmental medial release is undertaken. Before a deltoid release, it is imperative to remove any osteophytes on the tip of the medial malleolus, because their tenting effect shortens the deltoid. Palpation can reveal any discrete tight bands in the deep deltoid. If this procedure is insufficient, subperiosteal dissection of the deltoid ligament is undertaken until adequate release is achieved. This sequential release increases the resection gap and thereby the depth of the polyethylene insert. This technique highlights the importance of the accuracy of the depth of the distal tibial resection. If lateral ligament laxity is still present, the authors perform a lateral ligament reconstruction with a modification of the Chrisman-Snook procedure (Fig. 4) [94].

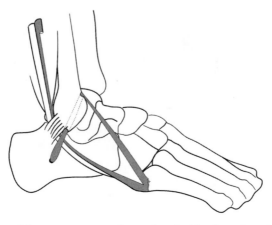

Fig. 4. Lateral ligament reconstruction as described by Acevedo and Myerson.

Management of associated problems when performing total ankle replacement

Assessments of alignment should include full clinical examination of the legs, together with radiographic assessment (Figs. 5 and 6). Deformity can arise above the ankle (eg, following tibial malunion), in the ankle (as a function of the degenerative process itself), or below the ankle in the foot (eg, from neuromuscular problems). Thus recognition and appropriate imaging are essential prerequisites to guide the treatment. The authors have found that weight-bearing full-length limb-alignment radiographs, in addition to standard ankle views, are useful and may unmask hitherto unrecognized deformity. (The authors now routinely obtain these radiographs before TAR.) They also suggest that forced weight-bearing dorsiflexion and plantar flexion views of the ankle be obtained. These views are extremely helpful in determining the arc of movement of the ankle and any relative hypermobility of the hindfoot. Anterior subluxation of the talus during the forced plantar flexion views also will heighten clinical suspicion of lateral ligament insufficiency as the talus rotates anteromedially around the functionally intact deltoid ligament. If the varus arises from a symptomatic varus arthritic knee, total knee arthroplasty should be undertaken before a TAR. Tibia vara or supramalleolar malalignment should be corrected before TAR surgery; the authors believe that correction of such a deformity combined with ankle arthroplasty would be excessive surgery for the patient's limb at one time.

Cavovarus deformity. The characteristics of the cavovarus foot predispose the patient to a varus ankle deformity and possibly degeneration. A wide spectrum of deformity exists, from the slightly deformed ankle to a severely deformed cavovarus foot and ankle with lateral ligament insufficiency and peroneus brevis weakness. Cavovarus deformity also has been reported to

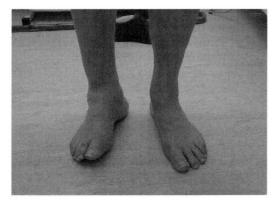

Fig. 5. Typical clinical appearance of an arthritic varus ankle.

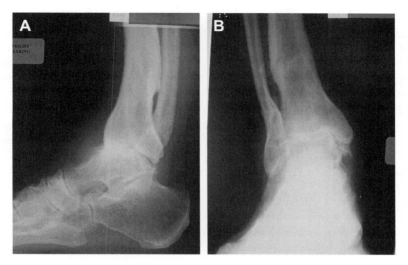

Fig. 6. (*A*, *B*) A varus deformed arthritic ankle secondary to tibial malunion.

be more frequent in patients who have lateral ankle instability, the former condition almost certainly predisposing the development of the latter [95]. Thus, when addressing the degenerate ankle in such a patient, one must be very conscious of the associated deformities:

- Contracted deltoid ligament
- Lateral ligament insufficiency
- Varus heel
- Focal medial bone loss
- Plantar flexion of the first metatarsal
- Medially displaced tendo Achilles

Assessment also must determine if the hindfoot deformity is fixed or flexible and thus direct the treatment appropriately. A fixed deformity alters the ankle biomechanics and will lead to arthritis [49]. Identification of the apex of the deformity is imperative. Is the deformity driven by the hindfoot, midfoot, forefoot, or a combination of all three? The Coleman block test will show the hindfoot varus to be corrected once the first ray is accommodated or, conversely, whether the hindfoot is flexible and driven by a plantar flexed first ray. It may be that a dorsiflexion osteotomy of the first metatarsal is all that is required to produce correction. The heel often remains in varus, however. In that case a lateral displacement calcaneal osteotomy also is required to minimize the varus moment about the ankle.

Additional procedures. Residual malalignment following TAR leads to instability, edge loading, and early failure. Therefore some authors consider such deformities to be contraindications to TAR [65], with 15° commonly being considered the upper limit for TAR [48]. Varus malalignment is a particular problem that can lead to a twofold increase in revision rate (Figs. 7 and 8) [96]. Thus additional procedures need to be considered to correct or address varus deformities if TAR is performed in such ankles. Additional soft tissue procedures include lateral ligament reconstruction, deltoid ligament release, tibialis tendon transfer, and peroneal tendon transfer.

There are several ways of carrying out lateral ligament reconstruction, as mentioned later. What must be remembered is to debride the lateral gutter of osteophytes and other structures to allow derotation of the talus back into the mortise.

Deltoid ligament release is performed from within the ankle. The deep portion is released first, and other portions are palpated and released as required while a corrective valgus force is applied to the ankle (Fig. 9). Occasionally, a separate posteromedial incision also is necessary to lengthen the tibialis posterior and flexor digitalis longus tendons.

Muscular imbalance also may require correction, particularly overactivity of the peroneus longus, which can be transferred to the peroneus brevis. Correction will reduce first ray plantar flexion and improve hind- and midfoot eversion, thereby correcting the ankle varus.

After these procedures, the alignment of the hindfoot indicates whether a calcaneal osteotomy is necessary. A calcaneal osteotomy is performed by making a lateral oblique incision behind the peroneal tendons (taking care to preserve the sural nerve), performing a lateral sliding osteotomy that translates the posterior fragment 5 to 10 mm laterally, and fixing it with one or two large, cannulated, partially threaded cancellous screws. This procedure may be combined with dorsal displacement for a fuller

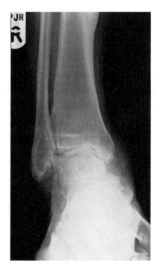

Fig. 7. Preoperative radiograph of a varus arthritic ankle.

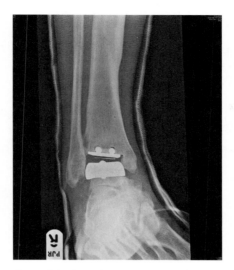

Fig. 8. Postoperative radiograph in the patient in Fig. 7. Inadequate soft tissue balancing and attempt to rectify varus with a valgus tibial cut will lead to early failure.

correction in the cavovarus foot [97]. If more correction is needed, a laterally based closing wedge is added [98].

Bony procedures include sliding osteotomy of the calcaneus, subtalar arthrodesis, and fibular shortening. Other bony techniques include a shortening fibular osteotomy (Fig. 10) and a medial malleolar osteotomy (see Fig. 3).

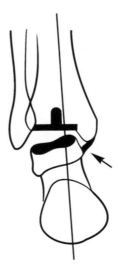

Fig. 9. Varus ankle with contracted medial/deltoid ligament.

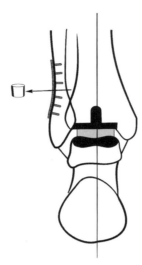

Fig. 10. Shortening fibular osteotomy.

Lateral ligament insufficiency/instability. Twenty-five percent to 30% of cases of ankle OA are thought to be associated with old lateral ligament ruptures that were not treated surgically. The radiographic appearance is typical. The hindfoot is in varus, the talus is tilted laterally and rotated internally, and the medial malleolus slopes to match the medial facet of the talus (Fig. 11) [99,100]. It has been suggested that ligament reconstruction

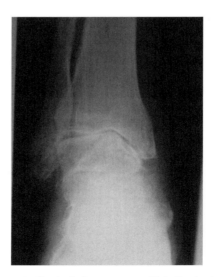

Fig. 11. Radiograph demonstrating typical appearances. Note the sloping medial malleolus and medial tibial erosion.

alone in patients who have mild degenerative disease can halt the progression of the disease [100], but there have been no definitive longitudinal studies. It is prudent to stabilize such ankles with a ligament reconstruction if TAR is being considered. This stabilization can be done before or at the time of the joint replacement surgery. Both anatomic (Broström) or non-anatomic (Chrisman-Snook) procedures have been described. Patients who have underlying muscle paralysis or imbalance giving abnormal ligamentous structure are better managed with arthrodesis, however. Cavovarus foot deformity also can be seen in patients who have chronic lateral ligamentous insufficiency in the absence of underlying neurologic abnormality. Such patients have been treated successfully by a combination of lateral displacement calcaneal osteotomy, modified Broström lateral ligament reconstruction, and dorsiflexion first metatarsal osteotomy, as required (Figs. 12 and 13) [49].

Hindfoot and knee arthritis. Associated arthritis of the hindfoot can present several decision-making dilemmas, depending on the amount of deformity and the symptoms related to the joint concerned. Isolated subtalar OA without deformity can be arthrodesed at the time of TAR if there is no danger of devascularising the talus. Alternatively, in cases of isolated subtalar OA, some authors advocate TAR alone, the rationale being that the subtalar joint becomes asymptomatic after TAR because it no longer is required to move to the same degree. When significant associated deformity requires a triple arthrodesis, it is better to perform this procedure before the TAR to avoid too much stripping of talus and thus incurring the risk of Avascular Necrosis (Figs. 14 and 15). Also, the prolonged casting required for healing

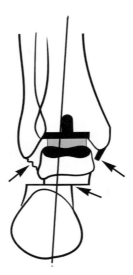

Fig. 12. Deltoid ligament release and medial displacement calcaneal osteotomy.

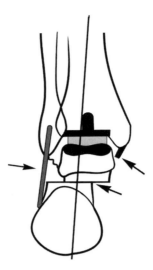

Fig. 13. Total ankle replacement plus medial release and non-anatomic ligament reconstruction.

of a hindfoot arthrodesis would result in poor movement of the ankle. Hence the accepted teaching is a staged procedure of single/triple arthrodesis of the affected joints followed 3 to 6 months later by TAR [101,102] or by either a tibio-talocalcaneal or pantalar arthrodesis, thereby avoiding potential problems with talar vascularity that may affect the structural integrity of the bone.

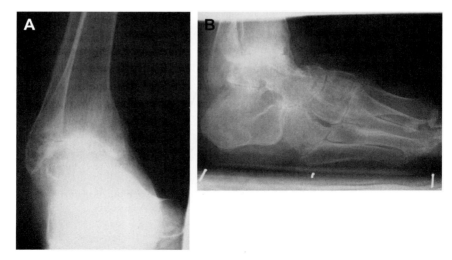

Fig. 14. (*A*, *B*) Preoperative radiographs of a varus ankle in a rheumatoid patient.

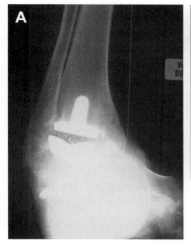
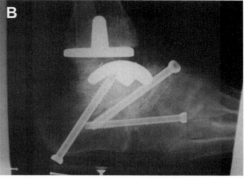

Fig. 15. (*A, B*) Radiographs of the patient in Fig. 14 4 months after total ankle replacement and corrective triple arthrodesis. The talus has collapsed with subsequent failure of the prosthesis. The patient was revised to a pantalar arthrodesis using an intramedullary nail.

Lower limb malalignment. For symptomatic knee arthritis, the generally accepted teaching is to address the knee first by a high tibial osteotomy or by unicompartmental or total knee replacement surgery, whichever is deemed most appropriate. A problem arises if the knee is asymptomatic but deformed. In this case, if an arthrodesis or TAR is performed in good alignment in a limb with a varus knee, the ankle will become valgus when the knee is subsequently realigned, with consequences for the prosthesis (if TAR is performed) or for the hind- and midfoot (if the ankle is arthrodesed).

In cases of tibial malunion, a supramalleolar or tibial osteotomy can be performed [5,7,103]. Although excellent or good results have been achieved, a proportion of patients require further surgery, either arthrodesis or TAR. Supramalleolar osteotomy allows further surgery to be performed successfully in a biomechanically corrected environment. For operative technique, see the review article by LaClair [104].

Recurrent deformity. If deformity recurs, it tends to happen after the patient begins weight bearing, because of intraoperative errors in estimating the weigh-bearing axis or because of dynamic muscle imbalance. Mild deformity can be addressed by physiotherapy, in cases of muscular weakness/atrophy or tendoachilles/gastrocnemius tightness, for which strengthening/stretching exercises are useful. Greater deformity requires further surgical intervention, usually to address factors that were present preoperatively but were addressed incompletely or not at the time of the primary procedure.

Summary

Treatment of the arthritic varus ankle presents a significant surgical challenge. The recognition of the causes and associated deformities directs treatment in the individual patient and optimizes functional outcome. Arthrodesis and TAR often need to be augmented by corrective hind- and midfoot procedures and by careful soft tissue balancing. Often multiple procedures are required to achieve the desired result, and patients need to be advised that surgery may need to be staged.

References

[1] Doets HC, van der Plaat LW, Klein JP. Medial malleolar osteotomy for the correction of varus deformity during total ankle arthroplasty: results in 15 ankles. Foot Ankle Int 2008; 29:171–7.

[2] Tochigi Y, Rudert MJ, Saltzman CL, et al. Contribution of articular surface geometry to ankle stabilization. J Bone Joint Surg Am 2006;88:2704–13.

[3] Benthien RA, Myerson MS. Supramalleolar osteotomy for ankle deformity and arthritis. Foot Ankle Clin 2004;9:475–87.

[4] Mangone PG. Distal tibial osteotomies for the treatment of foot and ankle disorders. Foot Ankle Clin 2001;6:583–97.

[5] Stamatis ED, Myerson MS. Supramalleolar osteotomy: indications and technique. Foot Ankle Clin 2003;8:317–33.

[6] Swords MP, Nemec S. Osteotomy for salvage of the arthritic ankle. Foot Ankle Clin 2007; 12:1–13.

[7] Takakura Y, Tanaka Y, Kumai T, et al. Low tibial osteotomy for osteoarthritis of the ankle. Results of a new operation in 18 patients. J Bone Joint Surg Br 1995;77:50–4.

[8] Takakura Y, Takaoka T, Tanaka Y, et al. Results of opening-wedge osteotomy for the treatment of a post-traumatic varus deformity of the ankle. J Bone Joint Surg Am 1998; 80:213–8.

[9] Tanaka Y, Takakura Y, Hayashi K, et al. Low tibial osteotomy for varus-type osteoarthritis of the ankle. J Bone Joint Surg Br 2006;88:909–13.

[10] Pagenstert GI, Hintermann B, Barg A, et al. Realignment surgery as alternative treatment of varus and valgus ankle osteoarthritis. Clin Orthop Relat Res 2007;462:156–8.

[11] Cheng YM, Huang PJ, Hong SH, et al. Low tibial osteotomy for moderate ankle arthritis. Arch Orthop Trauma Surg. 2001;121(6):355–8.

[12] Stamatis ED, Cooper PS, Myerson MS. Supramalleolar osteotomy for the treatment of distal tibial angular deformities and arthritis of the ankle joint. Foot Ankle Int 2003;24: 754–64.

[13] Hefti FL. Ankle joint fusion determination of optimal position by gait analysis. Arch Orthop Trauma Surg 1980;96:187–95.

[14] Thomas RH, Daniels TR. Ankle arthritis. J Bone Joint Surg Am 2003;85:923–36.

[15] Waters RL, Barnes G, Husserl T, et al. Comparable energy expenditures after arthrodesis of the hip and ankle. J Bone Joint Surg Am 1988;70:1032–7.

[16] Mann RA. Surgical implications of biomechanics of the foot and ankle. Clin Orthop Relat Res 1980;146:111–8.

[17] Morris JM. Biomechanics of the foot and ankle. Clin Orthop Relat Res 1977;122:10–7.

[18] Mazur JM, Schwartz E, Simon SR. Ankle arthrodesis. Long term follow-up with gait analysis. J Bone Joint Surg Am 1979;61:964–75.

[19] Morgan CD, Henke JA, Bailey RW, et al. Long-term results of tibiotalar arthrodesis. J Bone Joint Surg Am 1985;67:546–50.

[20] Buck P, Morrey BF, Chao EY. The optimum position of arthrodesis of the ankle. A gait study of the knee and ankle. J Bone Joint Surg Am 1987;69:1052–62.
[21] Helm R. The results of ankle arthrodesis. J Bone Joint Surg Br 1990;72:141–3.
[22] Scranton PE Jr, Fu FH, Brown TD. Ankle arthrodesis: a comparative clinical and biomechanical evaluation. Clin Orthop Relat Res 1980;151:234–43.
[23] Baciu CC. A simple technique for arthrodesis of the ankle. J Bone Joint Surg Br 1986;68: 266–7.
[24] Gallie WE. Arthrodesis of the ankle joint. J Bone Joint Surg Br 1948;30:619–21.
[25] Adams JC. Arthrodesis of the ankle joint. Experiences with the transfibular approach. J Bone Joint Surg Br 1948;30:506–11.
[26] Wilson HJ Jr. Arthrodesis of the ankle: a technique using bilateral hemimalleolar onlay grafts with screw fixation. J Bone Joint Surg Am 1969;51:775–7.
[27] Mäenpää H, Lehto MUK, Belt EA. Why do ankle arthrodeses fail in patients with rheumatic disease? Foot Ankle Int 2001;22:403–8.
[28] Holt ES, Hansen ST, Mayo KA, et al. Ankle arthrodesis using internal screw fixation. Clin Orthop Relat Res 1991;268:21–8.
[29] Maurer RC, Cimino WR, Cox CV, et al. Transarticular cross screw fixation. A technique of ankle arthrodesis. Clin Orthop Relat Res 1991;268:56–64.
[30] Mann RA, Van Manen JW, Wapner K, et al. Ankle fusion. Clin Orthop Relat Res 1991; 268:49–55.
[31] Cannon LB, Brown J, Cooke PH. Early weightbearing is safe following arthroscopic ankle arthrodesis. Foot Ankle Surg 2004;10:135–9.
[32] Scranton PE. Use of internal compression in arthrodesis of the ankle. J Bone Joint Surg Am 1985;67:550–5.
[33] Gruen GS, Mears DC. Arthrodesis of the ankle and subtalar joints. Clin Orthop Relat Res 1991;268:15–20.
[34] Sowa DT, Krackow KA. Ankle fusion: a new technique of internal fixation using a compression blade plate. Foot Ankle 1989;9:232–40.
[35] Weltmer JB Jr, Choi SH, Shenoy A, et al. Wolf blade plate ankle arthrodesis. Clin Orthop Relat Res 1991;268:107–11.
[36] Carrier DA, Harris CM. Ankle arthrodesis with vertical Steinmann's pins in rheumatoid arthritis. Clin Orthop Relat Res 1991;268:10–4.
[37] Kile TA, Donnelly RE, Gehrke JC, et al. Tibiotalocalcaneal arthrodesis with an intramedullary device. Foot Ankle Int 1994;15(12):669–73.
[38] Moore TJ, Prince R, Pochatko D, et al. Retrograde intramedullary nailing for ankle arthrodesis. Foot Ankle Int 1995;16:433–6.
[39] Charnley J. Compression arthrodesis of the ankle and shoulder. J Bone Joint Surg Br 1951; 33:180–91.
[40] Mission JR, Anderson JG, Bohay DR, et al. External fixation techniques for foot and ankle fusions. Foot Ankle Clin 2004;9:529–39.
[41] Myerson MS. Ankle arthrodesis. In: Reconstructive foot and ankle surgery. Philadelphia: Elsevier Saunders; 2005. p. 443–58.
[42] Stone JW. Arthroscopic ankle arthrodesis. Foot Ankle Clin 2006;11:361–8.
[43] Ferkel RD, Hewitt M. Long-term results of arthroscopic ankle arthrodesis. Foot Ankle Int 2005;26:275–80.
[44] Dent CM, Patil M, Fairclough JA. Arthroscopic ankle arthrodesis. J Bone Joint Surg Br 1993;75:830–2.
[45] Glick JM, Morgan MS, Myerson TG, et al. Ankle arthrodesis using an arthroscopic method: long term follow up of 34 cases. Arthroscopy 1996;12:428–34.
[46] Zvijac JE, Lemak L, Schurhoff MR, et al. Analysis of arthroscopically assisted ankle arthrodesis. Arthroscopy 2002;18(1):70–5.
[47] Turan I, Wredmark T, Fellander-Tsai L. Arthroscopic ankle arthrodesis in rheumatoid arthritis. Clin Orthop Relat Res 1995;320:110–4.

[48] Smith R, Wood PL. Arthrodesis of the ankle in the presence of a large deformity in the coronal plane. J Bone Joint Surg Br 2007;89:615–9.

[49] Fortin PT, Guettler J, Manoli A. Idiopathic cavovarus and lateral ankle instability: recognition and treatment implications relating to ankle arthritis. Foot Ankle Int 2002;23: 1031–7.

[50] Stroud CC. Arthroscopic arthrodesis of the ankle, subtalar, and first metatarsophalangeal joint. Foot Ankle Clin 2002;7:135–46.

[51] Myerson MS, Quill G. Ankle arthrodesis: a comparison of an arthroscopic and an open method of treatment. Clin Orthop Relat Res 1991;268:84–95.

[52] O'Brien TS, Hart TS, Shereff MJ, et al. Open versus arthroscopic ankle arthrodesis: a comparative study. Foot Ankle Int 1999;20(6):368–74.

[53] Ogilvie-Harris DJ, Lieberman I, Fitsialos D. Arthroscopically assisted arthrodesis for osteoarthritic ankles. J Bone Joint Surg Am 1993;75:1167–74.

[54] Winson I, Robinson DE, Allen PE. Arthroscopic ankle arthrodesis. J Bone Joint Surg Br 2005;87:343–7.

[55] Gougoulias NE, Agathangelidis FG, Parsons SW. Arthroscopic ankle arthrodesis. Foot Ankle Int 2007;28:695–706.

[56] Morrey BF, Wiedeman GP. Complications and long-term results of ankle arthrodesis following trauma. J Bone Joint Surg Am 1980;62:777–84.

[57] Cobb TK, Gabrielsen TA, Campbell DC II, et al. Cigarette smoking and non-union after ankle arthrodesis. Foot Ankle Int 1994;15(2):64–7.

[58] Kitaoka HB, Alexander IJ, Adelaar RS, et al. Clinical rating systems for the ankle-hindfoot, midfoot, hallux and lesser toes. Foot Ankle Int 1994;15(7):349–53.

[59] Haddad SL, Coetzee JC, Estok R, et al. Intermediate and long term outcomes of total ankle arthroplasty and ankle arthrodesis. A systemic review of the literature. J Bone Joint Surg Am 2007;89:1899–905.

[60] Baker PL. SACH heel improves results of ankle fusion. J Bone Joint Surg Am 1970;52: 1485–6.

[61] Michelson JD, Schmidt GR, Mizel MS. Kinematics of a total arthroplasty of the ankle: comparison to normal ankle motion. Foot Ankle Int 2000;21(4):278–84.

[62] Anderson T, Montgomery F, Carlsson A. Uncemented STAR total ankle prostheses: three to eight-year follow-up of fifty-one consecutive ankles. J Bone Joint Surg Am 2003;85: 1321–9.

[63] Knecht SI, Estin M, Callaghan J, et al. The Agility total ankle arthroplasty. Seven to sixteen-year follow-up. J Bone Joint Surg Am 2004;86:1161–71.

[64] San Giovanni TP, Keblish DJ, Thomas WH, et al. Eight-year results of a minimally constrained total ankle arthroplasty. Foot Ankle Int 2006;27(6):418–26.

[65] Wood PL, Deakin S. Total ankle replacement. The results in 200 ankles. J Bone Joint Surg Br 2003;85:334–41.

[66] Doets HC, van Middlekoop M, Houdijk H, et al. Gait analysis after successful mobile bearing total ankle replacement. Foot Ankle Int 2007;28(3):313–22.

[67] Valderrabano V, Nigg BM, von Tscharner V, et al. Total ankle replacement in ankle osteoarthritis: an analysis of muscle rehabilitation. Foot Ankle Int 2007;28(2):281–91.

[68] Gellman H, Lenihan M, Halikis N, et al. Selective tarsal arthrodesis: an in vitro analysis of the effect on foot motion. Foot Ankle 1987;8(3):127–33.

[69] Hintermann B, Nigg BM. Influence of arthrodeses on kinematics of the axially loaded ankle complex during dorsiflexion/plantarflexion. Foot Ankle Int 1995;16(10):633–6.

[70] Sealey RJ, Myerson MS, Molloy AP, et al. Range of motion of the hindfoot following ankle arthrodesis: a prospective analysis. In: Programme and presentation book of the Annual Scientific Meeting of the British Orthopaedic Foot and Ankle Society. 2007.

[71] Ahlberg A, Henricson AS. Late results of ankle fusion. Acta Orthop Scand 1981;52(1): 103–5.

[72] Coester LM, Saltzman CL, Leupold J, et al. Long-term results following ankle arthrodesis for post-traumatic arthritis. J Bone Joint Surg Am 2001;83:219–28.
[73] Kofoed H, Sturup J. Comparison of ankle arthroplasty and arthrodesis. A prospective series with long-term follow-up. Foot 1994;4:6–9.
[74] SooHoo NF, Zingmond DS, Ko CY. Comparison of reoperation rates following ankle arthrodesis and total ankle arthroplasty. J Bone Joint Surg Am 2007;89:2143–9.
[75] Greisberg J, Assal M, Flueckiger G, et al. Takedown of ankle fusion and conversion to total ankle replacement. Clin Orthop Relat Res 2004;424:80–8.
[76] Lord G, Marrotte JH. Total ankle prosthesis. Technique and first results. Apropos of 12 cases. Rev Chir Orthop Reparatrice Appar Mot 1973;59:139–51.
[77] Bonnin M, Judet T, Colombier JA, et al. Midterm results of the Salto total ankle prosthesis. Clin Orthop Relat Res 2004;424:6–18.
[78] Buechel FF Sr., Buechel FF Jr, Pappas MJ. Twenty-year evaluation of cementless mobile-bearing total ankle replacements. Clin Orthop Relat Res 2004;424:19–26.
[79] Doets HC, Brand R, Nelissen RG. Total ankle arthroplasty in inflammatory joint disease with the use of two mobile bearing designs. J Bone Joint Surg Am 2006;88:1272–84.
[80] Kofoed H. Scandinavian total ankle replacement (STAR). Clin Orthop Relat Res 2004;424: 73–9.
[81] Kopp FJ, Patel MM, Deland JT, et al. Total ankle arthroplasty with the agility prosthesis: clinical and radiographic evaluation. Foot Ankle Int 2006;27:97–103.
[82] Pyevich MT, Saltzman CL, Callaghan JJ, et al. Total ankle arthroplasty: a unique design. Two to twelve year follow-up. J Bone Joint Surg Am 1998;80:1410–20.
[83] Valderrabano V, Hintermann B, Dick W. Scandinavian total ankle replacement: a 3.7 year average follow up of 65 patients. Clin Orthop Relat Res 2004;424:47–56.
[84] Henricson A, Skoog A, Carlsson A. The Swedish ankle arthroplasty register: an analysis of 531 arthroplasties between 1993 and 2005. Acta Orthop 2007;78(5):569–74.
[85] Hosman AH, Mason RB, Hobbs T, et al. A New Zealand national joint registry review of 202 total ankle replacements followed for up to 6 years. Acta Orthop 2007;78(5): 584–91.
[86] Fevang BT, Lie SA, Havelin LI, et al. 257 ankle arthroplasties performed in Norway between 1994 and 2005. Acta Orthop 2007;78(5):575–83.
[87] Wood PL, Crawford LA, Suneja R, et al. Total ankle replacement for rheumatoid arthritis. Foot Ankle Clin 2007;12:497–508.
[88] Hobson S, Dhar S. Performance of total ankle replacements in ankles with significant pre-operative hind foot deformity. In: Programme and presentation book of the Annual Scientific Meeting of the British Orthopaedic Foot and Ankle Society. 2007.
[89] Haskell A, Mann RA. Ankle arthroplasty with preoperative coronal plane deformity. Short term results. Clin Orthop Relat Res 2004;424:98–103.
[90] Stauffer RN, Chao EY, Brewster RC. Force and motion analysis of the normal, diseased and prosthetic ankle joint. Clin Orthop Relat Res 1977;127:189–96.
[91] Seireg A, Arvikar RJ. The prediction of muscular load sharing and joint forces in the lower extremities during walking. J Biomech 1975;8(2):89–102.
[92] Kofoed H. Ankle arthroplasty: indications, alignment, stability and gain in mobility. In: Kofoed H, editor. Current status of ankle arthroplasty. Berlin: Springer Verlag; 1998. p. 16–21.
[93] Stamatis ED, Myerson MS. How to avoid specific complications of total ankle replacement. Foot Ankle Clin 2002;7:765–87.
[94] Acevedo JI, Myerson MS. Modification of the Chrisman-Snook technique. Foot Ankle Int 2000;21(2):154–5.
[95] Manoli A II, Graham B. The subtle cavus foot, "the underpronator", a review. Foot Ankle Int 2005;26:256–63.
[96] Henricson A, Agren P-H. Secondary surgery after total ankle replacement: the influence of preoperative hindfoot alignment. Foot Ankle Surg 2007;13(1):41–4.

[97] Sammarco GJ, Taylor R. Cavovarus foot treated with combined calcaneus and metatarsal osteotomies. Foot Ankle Int 2001;22(1):19–30.

[98] Sullivan RJ, Aronow MS. Different faces of the triple arthrodesis. Foot Ankle Clin 2002; 7(1):95–106.

[99] Kofoed H. Old lateral ligament ruptures, osteoarthritis and ankle arthroplasty. Presented at International Federation of Foot & Ankle Societies, San Francisco, September 12–14, 2002.

[100] Harrington KD. Degenerative arthritis of the ankle secondary to long-standing lateral ligament instability. J Bone Joint Surg Am 1979;61:354–61.

[101] Greisberg J, Hansen ST Jr. Ankle replacement: management of associated deformities. Foot Ankle Clin 2002;7:721–36.

[102] Myerson MS, Miller SD. Salvage after complications of total ankle arthroplasty. Foot Ankle Clinics 2002;7:191–206.

[103] Pearce MS, Smith MA, Savidge GF. Supramalleolar tibial osteotomy for haemophilic arthropathy of the ankle. J Bone Joint Surg Br 1994;76:947–50.

[104] LaClair SM. Reconstruction of the varus ankle from soft-tissue procedures with osteotomy through arthrodesis. Foot Ankle Clin 2007;12:153–76.

ELSEVIER
SAUNDERS

Foot Ankle Clin N Am
13 (2008) 443–470

FOOT AND
ANKLE CLINICS

Valgus Ankle Deformity and Arthritis

Eric M. Bluman, MD, PhD[a,b,*],
Christopher P. Chiodo, MD[c]

[a]*Division of Orthopaedic Surgery, Madigan Army Medical Center,
9040A Fitzsimmons Avenue, Tacoma, WA 98431, USA*
[b]*Uniformed Services University of the Health Sciences, 4301 Jones Bridge Road,
Bethesda, MD 20814, USA*
[c]*Department of Orthopaedic Surgery, Brigham Foot and Ankle Center, Brigham and Women's
Hospital, Suite 56, 1153 Centre Street, Boston, MA 02130, USA*

Overview of ankle arthritis with coronal-plane deformity

Most ankle arthritis is symmetric in that the medial and lateral portions of the joint space are affected equally, but asymmetric cases are seen frequently. Valgus malalignment of the ankle or hindfoot increases pressure over the lateral portion of the tibiotalar and talofibular joints. Accompanying the increased pressure on the lateral mortise is diminished pressure, or even distraction, at the medial side [1]. This altered force pattern leads to pain and cartilage degradation on the lateral side with accompanying actual or perceived enlargement of the medial joint space. Global degenerative joint disease eventually ensues [2]. Asymmetric arthritis with varus deformity is more common and is discussed elsewhere in this issue.

This article describes several conditions that may result in valgus ankle arthritis. The emphasis is on correction of pathology or deformity to prevent valgus arthritis from developing. The surgical techniques available for the treatment of this form of ankle arthritis once it develops are described also.

Anatomy/biomechanics

Maintaining a congruent ankle mortise in a normal anatomic alignment depends on the osseous anatomy, ligamentous support, and the integrity of the articular cartilage. A substantial disturbance of any one of these

* Corresponding author. Foot and Ankle Surgery, Madigan Army Medical Center, 9040A Fitzsimmons Avenue, Tacoma, WA 98431.
E-mail address: emb43@cornell.edu (E.M. Bluman).

1083-7515/08/$ - see front matter. Published by Elsevier Inc.
doi:10.1016/j.fcl.2008.04.008

components can disrupt the balance of forces and eventually the congruity of the ankle joint.

The anatomic and mechanical axes of the leg are essentially coincident. Although it is commonly represented as normal to the axis of the leg, anatomic studies have shown that the plafond actually is in 3° of valgus. Normal anatomic variants may have up to 10° of valgus angulation [3].

Generally, deformities in the coronal plane are tolerated better than those in the sagittal plane [4] because small deformities in the coronal plane may be accommodated by subtalar motion (Fig. 1) [5]. Stiffness in the subtalar joint therefore may decrease the ability of the hindfoot to buffer focal tibiotalar contact pressures resulting from angular deformities of the tibia [2]. In fact, a frank loss of subtalar motion with a malpositioned surgical arthrodesis may cause the congruence of the mortise to be lost [6–8].

A number of retrospective studies have shown that patients who have longstanding valgus angulation at or above the tibiotalar joint do not develop substantial ankle arthritis [9,10]. The lack of longitudinal follow-up in these studies calls their clinical validity into question, however. Furthermore, retrospective studies looking at patients either with or without tibiotalar arthritis following joint malalignment carry a large risk of selection bias. As a result, these cohorts may be composed of patients that have been selected for their resistance to developing ankle arthrosis for one reason or another. Factors proposed to explain the difficulty of conducting longitudinal studies on this patient population include the slow progression of

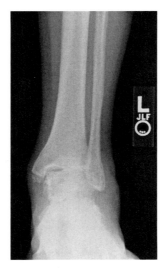

Fig. 1. Valgus ankle deformity being compensated by varus hindfoot. Note that the hindfoot has assumed a compensatory varus position to maintain the calcaneus along the weight-bearing axis of the leg. Note also the incompetence of the deltoid ligament.

the disease, patients' poor tolerance of deformity, and the ready availability of treatments [11]. Despite the lack of uniform clinical evidence to support realignment surgery, some authors have recommended surgical correction for distal tibial deformity as little as 5° [12,13].

Unlike the clinical studies demonstrating minimal joint degradation from coronal-plane deformity, basic science studies have revealed multiple adverse effects of malalignment. Critical amounts of tibiotalar joint angulation cause joint contact areas to decrease by 10% or more [4,5,14]. Abnormal pressure patterns within a joint cause localized cartilage wear and production of debris [15] and also lead to edema in the subchondral bone [16]. The presence of articular debris within the joint generates synovitis [17,18]. Together, these effects promote a positive feedback loop driving further joint degradation and causing or worsening deformity.

Even small amounts of fibular displacement, shortening, or rotational deformity have profound effects on the pressures experienced within the lateral ankle joint [19]. Numerous studies have demonstrated that the fibula functions both in buttressing the lateral joint and in load transmission [20,21] Loss of this modest but important weight-bearing function places increased pressure on the lateral plafond with eventual cartilage damage and potential subsidence of distal tibial bone. Valgus angulation may ensue. These findings have prompted some to suggest that any deformity of the fibula requires anatomic restoration to avoid the possibility of later joint degradation [19,22].

In most patients a small amount of valgus angulation at the plafond is well tolerated [9,10]. The problem in many cases is not the presence of a small static deformity but rather the progression of valgus angulation. The presence of intact cortical bone in the lateral distal tibia is an important factor in preventing this progression. Aitken and colleagues [23] demonstrated that the subchondral bone of the tibial plafond has an elastic modulus between 300 and 450 MPa, but removal of the subchondral cortex reduces the ability of the underlying bone to resist compression forces by 30% to 50%. The resistance to compressive forces diminishes proximally until it virtually disappears 3 cm from the plafond. It follows from these findings that, once the biomechanical integrity of the subchondral bone of the lateral plafond is compromised, further valgus angulation will occur if corrective action is not taken.

The medial ligamentous structures and the lateral malleolar buttress complement each other in preventing lateral translation and valgus angulation of the talus. Either can prevent lateral translation, at least temporarily. Supination external rotation (SER) ankle injuries illustrate this point. The second stage of SER injuries is characterized by distal fibular fracture without disruption of the deltoid ligament or medial malleolus. After such an injury an external rotation or laterally directed force does not result in lateral translation of the talus despite the loss of the fibular buttress because of the intact deltoid ligament. In contrast, the SER type IV fracture variant with deltoid ligament disruption allows lateral translation of the talus. Surgical reduction and fixation of the lateral malleolus in these injuries restores congruity of the mortise and prevents lateral translation even without direct repair of the deltoid ligament [24].

The loss of the buttressing function of the lateral malleolus through its anchorage to the distal tibia also illustrates this point. In the case of syndesmosis disruption, the talus will not angulate into valgus or translate laterally as long as the deltoid ligament remains intact [25]. In the absence of deltoid ligament insufficiency, failure to restore and heal this lateral buttress through syndesmosis fixation leads to valgus angulation and/or lateral translation of the talus. A clinical case demonstrating an accelerated course of this situation is illustrated in Fig. 2.

The final stage of adult-acquired flatfoot deformity (AAFD) demonstrates that the bony architecture of the mortise alone is not adequate to prevent valgus deformity of the ankle in the chronic absence of medial ligamentous restraint. In stage IV AAFD the lateral buttress function of the fibula is intact, but constant tensile forces on the deltoid and capsular complexes caused by longstanding hindfoot valgus lead to increased strain and eventual talar valgus angulation. This angulation is followed by edge loading of the lateral talus and lateral articular degradation as the talus is "levered" out of the mortise. The increased pressure on the talofibular articulation even may result in a fibular stress fracture [26].

Mechanisms of developing valgus ankle deformity and arthritis

Although valgus ankle arthritis is not encountered as commonly as other forms of ankle arthritis, it may result from a number of conditions (Box 1). Fractures of the ankle can lead easily to immediate chondral damage, which over time may be compounded further by residual valgus deformity. Ankle fractures caused by three different mechanisms, each of which can lead to valgus deformity, are discussed in this article. Other conditions leading to valgus deformity are described thereafter.

Supination-external rotation ankle fractures

In grades II through IV of the SER ankle fracture classification system, the fibula may demonstrate shortening, external rotation, and/or angulation. Any of these deformities may predispose the development of increased pressure within the lateral joint. The most common pattern is a combination of shortening and external rotation of the distal fibular fragment [27]. SER fractures that malunite with shortening and external rotation of the fibula may allow lateral rotation and abduction of the talus. Even with maintenance of deltoid ligament integrity, the loss of lateral joint congruence and fibular support places increased pressure on the lateral plafond. Not surprisingly, chronic malunions eventually develop lateral ankle joint arthrosis.

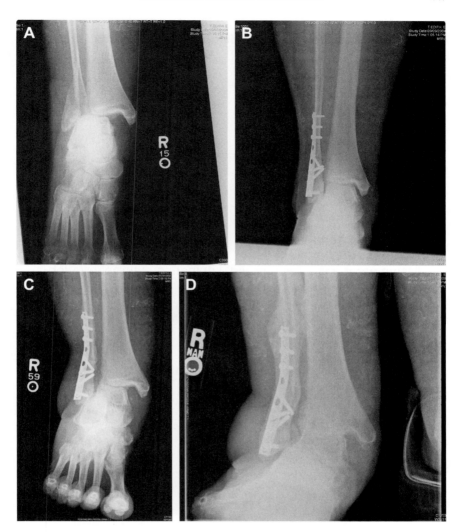

Fig. 2. Development of asymmetric tibiotalar valgus arthritis as a result of unrecognized syndesmosis disruption in conjunction with deltoid ligament rupture in a neuropathic diabetic patient. Anteroposterior roentgenograms of ankle fracture associated with syndesmotic injury and deltoid ligament disruption at time of (A) injury and (B) reduction and plating of fibular fracture without fixation of distal tibiofibular syndesmosis. (C) By 4 months after open reduction and internal fixation there is further subluxation of the talus and asymmetric degeneration of the tibial plafond. (D) Sixteen months after open reduction and internal fixation the patient presented to the first author's office with such severe valgus degeneration that joint salvage was impossible, and tibiotalocalcaneal fusion was necessary. It is possible that fusion could have been avoided with initial reduction and fixation using multiple syndesmotic screws followed by a prolonged period of enforced non–weight bearing.

Box 1. Causes of valgus ankle deformity and arthritis

Pediatric conditions
  Fibular shortening
  Poliomyelitis
  Spina bifida
  Cerebral palsy
  Pseudoarthrosis of fibula
  Vascularized free fibular transfer
  Hereditary multiple exostosis
  Multiple epiphyseal dysplasias
  Morquio syndrome
  Clubfoot residua

Sequelae of trauma
  Malunion of pilon fracture
  Malunion of ankle fracture (eg, supination external rotation
    or pronation-abduction types)
  Malunion distal tibial fracture
  Improperly reduced syndesmosis disruption

Degenerative conditions
  Rheumatoid arthritis
  Stage IV adult-acquired flatfoot deformity
  Tarsal coalition

Other
  Hemophilic arthropathy
  Charcot neuroarthropathy
  Failure of total ankle arthroplasty

Pronation-abduction ankle fractures

The pronation-abduction ankle fracture pattern within the Lauge-Hansen classification system is uncommon, accounting for a small minority of rotational injuries [28]. This fracture type can be difficult to treat because of fibular comminution and the impaction of the lateral tibial plafond by the talus [29]. Improper restoration of the fibular length and alignment as well as failure to disimpact and stabilize the lateral plafond can predispose the affected ankle to valgus deformity and eventual arthritis.

Anatomic reduction and fixation of these fractures minimizes the chance of developing deformity and subsequent arthritis. Limbird and Aaron [29] presented a series of patients who had sustained pronation-abduction ankle fractures. In this series, reduction of the medial malleolus was performed initially to allow reduction and stabilization of the talus beneath the plafond.

Fibular length, rotation, and angulation were corrected subsequently in an open manner using the lateral aspect of the talus as a template. Contoured plating then was used to fix the reduction. Bone grafting was used in six of eight patients and resulted in union of all those fibulae. Fractures that did not receive primary bone grafting went on to non-union and subsequently required secondary grafting procedures to obtain union [29]. More recently, Siegel and Tornetta [28] presented an extraperiosteal method to plate and reduce the fibula in pronation-abduction injuries. All fractures in their series went on to heal without displacement.

Pilon fracture

Pilon fractures, particularly those with total articular involvement (Arbeitsgemeinshaft für Osteosynthesefragen [AO] type C), are at risk for malunion. In a study of 145 pilon fractures treated with a variety of techniques, almost one fifth were judged to suffer from malunion [30]. Teeny and Wiss [31] treated 60 pilon fractures with internal fixation and found that those with a Reudi type III (AO type C) pattern were seven times more likely to be complicated by malunion. Patterns in which the fibula remains intact have a propensity to drift into varus, whereas those with fibular involvement may develop valgus deformity if not anatomically reduced and fixed.

Anatomic reduction and stable fixation of the fibula may be the most important step in reconstruction of these fractures to ensure that there is not subsequent valgus malunion. Tile [32] counseled, "Failure to reconstruct the fibula at all is a major error in judgment and may jeopardize the tibial reconstruction, as the tendency of the ankle to drift into valgus will be difficult to overcome." Aided by talofibular and tibiotalar articular congruity as well as ligamentotaxis, the Chaput fragment frequently reduces into a nearly anatomic position with restoration of fibular length and alignment [33]. Restoration of the fibular osseous anatomy in this way can allow later definitive surgical fixation by preventing contracture of the soft tissues as their condition improves. For definitive fixation of the distal tibia, the authors have found the newly developed contoured-locking plates are effective in preventing recurrence of deformity once the fracture has been reduced anatomically. Early plating of the fibula has significant implications for the use of an anterolateral approach, particularly if the fibular fixation is done by a surgeon other than the one who will perform the definitive fixation. If early fibular reduction and fixation is considered necessary, the surgeon performing this step needs to coordinate the location of the incision with the surgeon who will be performing the definitive fixation.

Adult-acquired flatfoot deformity

AAFD usually manifests with deformity of the hindfoot and midfoot. The most advanced stage of AAFD (stage IV), however, occurs when severe hindfoot valgus eventually causes attenuation and failure of the deltoid ligament complex [26]. Deltoid incompetence allows valgus angulation of the talus within the mortise. Impingement of the lateral talus on the lateral plafond and distal fibula results from this angulation (Fig. 3). If allowed to continue, this impingement may eventually cause a stress fracture of the fibula.

If diagnosed early, the tibiotalar joint in stage IV AAFD remains supple and is reducible. With late diagnosis the joint frequently is irreducible, and there may be loss of lateral tibiotalar and/or talofibular joint space. The distinction between a reducible and irreducible tibiotalar joint distinguishes stage IVA disease from stage IVB disease and has implications for treatment [34]. With stage IVA disease, restoration of tibiotalar joint congruency is possible. In these patients surgical efforts should focus on tibiotalar joint–sparing procedures that involve restoration of foot alignment and reconstruction of the deltoid complex.

Cases of stage III AAFD that are undercorrected by previous triple arthrodesis may lead to a specialized form of the disease. These patients may present with tibiotalar valgus angulation and, frequently, with some valgus ankle arthritis (Fig. 4). The residual valgus hindfoot places a large tensile force on the medial ligamentous complex [7,8]. This force results in ligament strain and eventually incompetence. Here, again, the end result is a valgus tibiotalar incongruity [6]. Treatment options for the different forms of valgus ankle arthritis caused by AAFD are reviewed later.

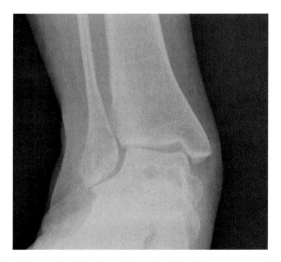

Fig. 3. Stage IVA adult-acquired flat foot deformity. Standing anteroposterior roentgenogram of patient demonstrating deltoid ligament insufficiency secondary to severe, long-standing hindfoot valgus.

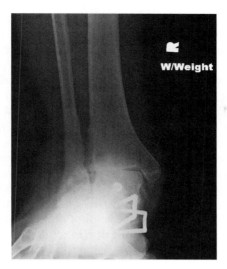

Fig. 4. Valgus ankle arthritis secondary to under-corrected triple arthrodesis. Because of residual hindfoot valgus, the deltoid ligament complex becomes insufficient, and the talus tilts into valgus within the mortise.

Hemophilia

It is common for patients who have bleeding diastheses to experience hemarthroses. These hemarthroses occur spontaneously in patients who have severe hemophilia, which is defined as 1% or less of the normal level of functional circulating clotting factor (eg, factor VIII or IX) [35]. Hemarthroses are painful and destructive, especially if recurrent. The ankle is the third most commonly affected joint in the body [36]. Repeated ankle hemarthroses caused by any of the bleeding diastheses may lead to characteristic changes at the ankle and hindfoot. These changes include plantarflexion contracture, varus hindfoot, and valgus ankle arthritis. Factor replacement therapy helps prevent or limit hemarthroses, thereby preventing or delaying the development of hemophilic arthropathies. Unfortunately, patients may experience a downward-spiraling clinical course in which repeated bleeds lead to degeneration of the joint, increasing the need for factor replacement. Eventually the increased factor replacement becomes ineffective. The recommended treatment of hemophilic arthropathy of the ankle traditionally has been arthrodesis [36,37]. More recently, however, supramalleolar osteotomy has shown promise in slowing the progression of hemophilic arthropathy [38].

Pediatric disorders

The alignment of the ankle joint is dynamic throughout ontogeny. The fetal ankle is aligned in valgus. At the time of birth the valgus angulation measures about 10°. This valgus angulation decreases in early life until the ankle joint lies normal to the tibial axis by age 10 years [39].

A number of neuromuscular diseases that present in early childhood predispose a person to a valgus malaligned ankle. Dias [40] analyzed 100 anteroposterior roentgenograms of normal children at different ages. He found that in the normal child the distal fibular physis is 2 to 3 mm proximal to the dome of the talus during the first 4 years of life. Between 4 and 8 years of age the physis is at the same level as the talar dome. After this time, the physis resides 2 to 3 mm distal to the talar dome.

In the second part of the study, ankle roentgenograms of 173 pediatric patients who had obvious fibular shortening were analyzed. Most of these cases were caused by myelomeningocele. Other causes included poliomyelitis, cerebral palsy, fibular pseudarthrosis, and hereditary multiple osteochondromatosis. In all cases fibular shortening was associated with weakness of the soleus muscle, and the degree of fibular shortening was correlated with the magnitude of muscle weakness. Dias [40] hypothesized that the decreased downward pull of the fibular physis by the impaired soleus results in less stimulation of the physis and subsequent fibular shortening. There was no evidence of arthritis even with severe fibular shortening, probably because of the young age of this population.

The presence of open physes allows the development of angular deformities during childhood. Once a valgus deformity is initiated at the ankle, it is likely to progress until the physes fuse. The increased pressure imparted to the lateral portion of the ankle joint with valgus malalignment slows growth in the overlying physis, thereby leading to worsening of the deformity. Conditions leading to fibular shortening set this process in motion because they decrease or eliminate the proportion of weight borne by this bone and increase that seen at the lateral tibial physis. Injuries to the physis may result in asymmetric growth and valgus deformity.

Poliomyelitis

Although polio largely has been eliminated in the United States and the developed world, it remains endemic in a few countries. At its peak in the early 1950s there were 35,000 cases per year just in the United States. This incidence decreased to 2000 reported cases worldwide in 2006. Presently an estimated 600,000 individuals in the United States have residual health problems related to polio infection [41]. In 1965 Makin [42] reported on ankle alignment in 112 patients suffering from the late effects of poliomyelitis with asymmetric involvement of the lower extremities. In 87 of these patients shortening of the fibula was greater than that of the tibia. In addition to the shortened fibula, the distal tibial epiphysis had become deformed. The distal tibia had become a wedge with its base medial and apex lateral. The valgus deformity present was not caused by differential growth of the physis, because the growth plate remained intact and horizontal.

Hereditary multiple osteochondromatosis

Hereditary multiple osteochondromatosis is an autosomal dominant disorder in which multiple osteochondromas form along the metaphyses of long bones. Because the osteochondromas are associated with the physes, angular deformity or discrepancies in limb length may result. Approximately 50% of those who have the disease have ankle involvement, and in patients who have ankle involvement, a valgus deformity usually is observed (Fig. 5) [43]. Valgus deformities at the ankle result from fibular shortening and relative growth retardation of the lateral distal tibial physis [40,44].

Noonan and colleagues [43] studied 38 patients who had hereditary multiple osteochondromatosis who never had undergone any corrective surgery for deformity of the lower extremity. The average age of the group was 42 years. Sixty-seven percent of the cohort had a valgus ankle deformity. Of the 75 ankles evaluated (one was excluded because of previous open reduction and internal fixation), 19% showed radiographic evidence of degenerative joint disease. The joint deformity was significantly greater in the subjects who had degenerative joint disease than in those who did not have arthritic changes. Patients more than 40 years old had statistically less joint deformity than those younger than 40 years, suggesting that lesser degrees of joint angulation may develop degenerative changes with progression of time. The authors believe their findings suggest that prophylactic surgery to improve ankle alignment may be justified. They also cautioned that even more patients in their cohort may develop arthritic changes, because the average age at the time of the study was relatively low. The relatively

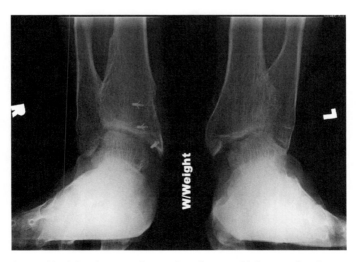

Fig. 5. Valgus ankle deformity secondary to hereditary multiple osteochondromatosis. Note the fibular shortening in addition to the valgus angulation at the tibial plafond on this antero-posterior roentgenogram of the bilateral ankles.

high percentage of patients who had ankle joint alignment deformities demonstrating arthritic changes is in contradistinction to studies that failed to show arthritis in patients who had other angular deformities [9].

Valgus deformity after total ankle arthroplasty

Although valgus deformity after total ankle arthroplasty (TAA) is technically not arthritis, the condition is listed here because some of the biomechanical concepts on which surgical correction are based are the same as those used with valgus ankle arthritis. Loss of coronal alignment after implantation is a known complication of TAA (Fig. 6) [45,46]. A common cause of this complication is intraoperative laceration or rupture of the deltoid ligament complex when cutting the medial tibia for component placement. Intraoperative or postoperative fracture of the medial malleolus also is a cause of failure of the medial restraints and eventual valgus tilt (Fig. 7). Finally, collapse of either the talar or tibial components can result in valgus malalignment of the weight-bearing axis. Regardless of cause, valgus malalignment of the TAA eventually results in edge loading and failure of the implant.

Patterns of valgus ankle deformity and arthritis

The authors are aware of only one previously published classification system for ankle arthritis associated with coronal deformity. This system

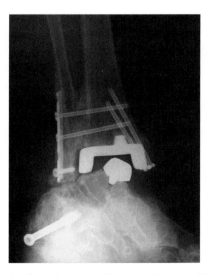

Fig. 6. Severe valgus edge loading of a total ankle arthroplasty resulting from deltoid ligament incompetence. Both the tibial and the talar components appear well fixed and are well aligned at their respective interfaces. (*Courtesy of* S. Raikin, MD, Philadelphia, PA.)

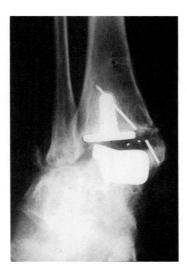

Fig. 7. Valgus deformity of total ankle arthroplasty resulting from intraoperative fracture of medial malleolus. Fixation placed at the time of fracture failed with resultant diastasis. Valgus subsidence of the tibial component ensued. (*From* Doets HC, Brand R, Nelissen RGHH. Total ankle arthroplasty in inflammatory disease with use of two mobile-bearing designs. J Bone Joint Surg 2006:88A:1277; with permission.)

organizes ankle arthritis into four categories: valgus congruent, valgus incongruent, varus congruent, and varus incongruent. An arthritic ankle was considered congruent if the tibiotalar joint convergence angle was less than 10°. Ankles with a greater amount of misalignment were defined as incongruent [47]. This classification system was developed to evaluate a cohort of patients about to undergo TAA. Although useful for this purpose, it is not applicable to all forms of valgus ankle arthritis.

From the previous discussion of causes of valgus ankle malalignment and arthritis, it is clear that a number of patterns of deformity may be observed. If substantial arthritic change associated with the deformity precludes salvage, the pattern of malalignment will not change if arthrodesis can be performed; the operative plan must ensure that a solid, well-aligned fusion is obtained. Alternatively, if TAA is to be used, the malalignment influences the soft tissue balancing that must be incorporated into the operative plan. If joint-sparing surgery is to be used, identification of the specific pattern of ankle deformity is crucial to obtain satisfactory results.

To this end the authors have devised a classification system (Table 1) based on the pathoanatomy present to help the orthopedic surgeon differentiate between patterns of deformity that may be encountered and to aid in choosing the proper joint-sparing surgery for each condition. It is organized primarily with respect to the locus of the deformity and secondarily with respect to the difficulty in obtaining a joint-sparing correction. Types I

Table 1
Classification system for patterns of valgus ankle deformity

Classification type	I	II	III	IV	V
Description	Supramalleolar deformity	Fibular shortening and distal tibial epiphyseal wedging	Fibular malunion; degradation of lateral articular surface	Impaction of lateral tibial plafond	Deltoid complex insufficiency with lateral edge loading
Cause	Pilon malunion or malunion of a distal tibia-fibula fracture	Poliomyelitis, cerebral palsy, or myelomeningocele	Unreduced/ malreduced SER ankle fracture	B- or C-type pilon malunion or malunion of a PA ankle fracture	Stage IVA AAFD
Joint-sparing surgical treatment	Supramalleolar osteotomy	Supramalleolar osteotomy with fibular lengthening	Correction of malreduction ± osteotomies to realign joint contact forces	Osteotomy for reduction and fixation of lateral plafond ± osteotomies to realign joint contact forces	Restoration of plantigrade foot with reconstruction of the deltoid ligament

Abbreviations: AAFD, adult-acquired flatfoot disorder; PA, pronation-abduction; SER, supination external rotation.

and II have deformity that will lead to valgus arthritis if left untreated. These deformities originate above the plafond. Types III and IV involve intra-articular damage that worsens with continued weight bearing if not corrected. The deformity of type V is initiated by intra- and extra-articular ligamentous insufficiency that is driven by foot pathology. The specific conditions named as leading to each of these forms of valgus ankle arthritis are only examples. The list is not exhaustive, and additional causes for the development of each form may be possible.

Because subfibular impingement may be encountered in each of these deformities, the integrity of the lateral ankle ligaments must be determined. Ligament repairs or reconstructions may be warranted as part of the joint-sparing surgical plan. Similarly the deltoid ligament complex may be intact or insufficient, with the exception of type V deformity in which the deltoid is necessarily insufficient. The integrity of the syndesmosis also should be evaluated before a treatment plan is finalized.

In type I malalignment the deformity originates from the supramalleolar region. The overall relationship of the mortise and talus is generally maintained, but the mechanical loading is shifted to the lateral part of the plafond and fibula. Occasionally the fibula may be shortened and malrotated relative to the talus. It may result from a valgus malunion of a pilon or distal tibiofibular fracture, by lateral distal tibial physeal arrest, or by hereditary multiple osteochondromatosis. The fibula may maintain a proper length and orientation relative to the talus or may be shortened. Joint-sparing surgery should consist of correction of the deformity with a supramalleolar osteotomy with lengthening of the fibula as required.

The type II valgus deformity develops in childhood from a variety of conditions. This pattern demonstrates fibular shortening with subsequent wedging of the lateral distal tibial epiphysis. The distal tibial physis does not show substantial angulation. Once the deformity is established, however, the increased lateral and decreased medial joint contact pressures may contribute through angular growth at the physis. Conditions that may lead to type II deformity include poliomyelitis, cerebral palsy, myelomeningocele, prior fibular harvesting for free transfer, and congenital pseudarthrosis of the fibula. In most of these conditions soleus weakness contributes to the growth retardation of the fibula. If treatment is undertaken before skeletal maturity, transphyseal closing osteotomy of the distal tibia with fibular-lengthening osteotomy may be attempted [48]. If treatment is delayed until after physeal closure, a distal tibial closing wedge osteotomy with fibular osteotomy should be used.

A third form occurs with selective loss of the lateral ankle joint cartilage with or without erosion of lateral subchondral bone. In the authors' experience this is the most common form of valgus arthritis. Here the overall weight-bearing axis of the tibia is unchanged, but the mechanical loading shifts pressure to the lateral part of the plafond and fibula. Congruency at the superior dome of the talus may be maintained if there is a gradual subsidence of the subchondral bone of the plafond or erosion of the cartilage, but there will be a loss of congruence at either the medial or lateral gutters or at both. Failure to reduce or maintain a reduction of a supination external rotation ankle fracture leads to decreased load being borne by the fibula and resultant increased pressure at the lateral joint (Fig. 8). Joint-sparing treatment, if possible, should include correction of the malunion, no matter how long standing it is [27]. Addition of an osteotomy (eg, calcaneal) to off-load the areas of damaged cartilage also may be required to minimize progression of arthritis.

In type IV deformity there is impaction of the lateral tibial plafond so that the congruency of the joint is disrupted. If there is associated fibular malalignment, the talus eventually may adopt a valgus position relative to the tibia. If the fibula is anatomic, there will be increased pressure at the apex of the plafond deformity with linear wear on the talar dome. This deformity may be seen in malunion of AO type B or C pilon fractures as well as with pronation-abduction ankle fractures (Fig. 9). Surgical correction of type IV deformities can be very difficult, because the compacted lateral plafond may involve a portion or the entire anteroposterior diameter of the plafond. Acute compaction of the lateral plafond (as may be seen in pronation-abduction injuries) may result in loss of congruence along the superior articular surface.

A fifth form occurs when the medial ligamentous restraints of the ankle joint become insufficient, allowing valgus tilting of the talus within the mortise. An example of this condition is stage IV AAFD in which the deltoid

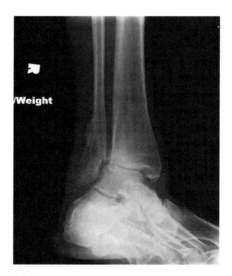

Fig. 8. Valgus ankle arthritis secondary to malunion of supination external rotation pattern ankle fracture. Mortise view demonstrating malunion of fibular fracture with shortening and external rotation, lateralization of talus within the mortise, and loss of lateral joint space.

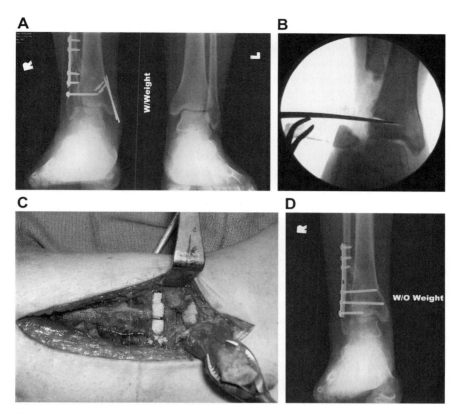

Fig. 9. Valgus malunion with fibular shortening of the fibula in an AO type C pilon consistent with type IV valgus deformity. (*A*) Roentgenogram obtained at presentation 4 months after the injury and initial surgery. Inadequate reduction and fixation was performed at initial surgery. (*B*) Intraoperative fluoroscopy of plafond at time of osteoclasis demonstrating osteotome being used to lever down the lateral plafond to re-establish a congruent articular surface. Fibular turndown osteotomy was used to gain access to plafond. (*C*) Intraoperative image demonstrating allograft placed within distal lateral tibial osteotomy site. Lengthening was performed before fixation of fibula and syndesmosis. (*D*) Despite marked improvement in deformity, the postoperative anteroposterior roentgenogram shows slight loss of reduction and recurrence of type IV deformity. It is possible that loss of reduction could have been avoided with placement of anterolateral distal tibial locking plate or by locking one third of the tubular plate on the fibula.

ligaments are rendered incompetent from excessive tensile loading secondary to a valgus hindfoot. Congruency of the ankle joint is no longer maintained, as may be noted first at the medial gutter and/or medial shoulder of the talar dome (see Fig. 2). Edge loading of the lateral talar dome on the lateral plafond occurs resulting in lateral articular degradation. This form leads to joint incongruity and subsequent valgus arthrosis if the foot deformity is not corrected in conjunction with ligamentous reconstruction.

Treatment

The treatment of valgus ankle arthritis always needs to be customized to the patient. A cookbook approach in which each patient who has valgus arthritis receives the same plan of care will result in frequent clinical failure. The surgeon needs to evaluate and consider several factors including, but not limited to, patient desires and expectations, comorbidities, the severity of arthritis, and the pattern of degenerative change. The patient who has valgus ankle arthritis may have one or more of the following conditions: contracted lateral ankle ligaments, deltoid ligament insufficiency, valgus hindfoot, shortened or deformed fibula, contracted heel cord, spring ligament insufficiency, or posterior tibialis insufficiency. Any of these pathologies, if present, needs to be addressed in the treatment plan.

Conservative treatments

Havenhill and colleagues [49] compared the effects of a University of California Biomechanics Laboratory (UCBL) orthosis with a medializing calcaneal osteotomy in a cadaveric adult acquired flatfoot model. This group found that both conditions significantly decreased the global mean contact pressures at the tibiotalar joint. The UCBL orthosis had a significantly greater effect on pressure normalization than the osteotomy. Reduction in peak contact pressure was reduced significantly from that observed in the flatfoot model when the UCBL orthosis was used. Clinical translation of these laboratory results may be limited, however. The cadaver model depended on a freely mobile subtalar joint. It is common for patients who have valgus ankle arthritis to have limited or absent subtalar motion. In addition, many clinicians have found that the UCBL orthosis is poorly tolerated. Because of problems with patient compliance, the authors choose to use custom-made semirigid orthoses rather than UCBLs.

Surgical treatments

A difficult question that may arise when considering tibiotalar joint salvage rather than arthrodesis in treating a patient who has valgus ankle arthritis is how much joint deterioration is acceptable. Unfortunately, there are no good clinical or radiographic signs to indicate that joint-sparing surgery will have a good chance of success. Re-establishment of hindfoot and mortise alignment in patients who have moderate-to-severe arthrosis may lessen pressure and relieve pain over the lateral joint line [13] but may overload the medial side because of changes in surface contact area [50,51]. Nevertheless, further long-term clinical research is necessary to determine just how much lateral degeneration is acceptable for joint salvage.

An argument may be made for performing a fusion at the index procedure to avoid potential deterioration of the medial tibiotalar articular cartilage that may occur with joint-sparing reconstruction of the deformity. The decision to fuse should be made only after considering all surgical alternatives and discussing these alternatives fully with the patient. Another option is to realign the weight-bearing axis with a hindfoot procedure and to perform a TAA if there is substantial progression of the tibiotalar arthritis. Although this treatment plan seems to provide a good option for patients who have moderate-to-severe valgus ankle arthritis, it should be entered into carefully.

Arthrodesis

Arthrodesis remains the reference standard for treating end-stage tibiotalar arthritis in patients with and without alignment abnormalities. Both short- and long-term studies have been reported in patients treated with open or arthroscopically aided procedures.

A handful of studies have reported on the long-term outcomes of ankle fusion. Coester and colleagues [52] reviewed a cohort of 23 patients who had undergone ankle arthrodesis. The mean follow-up for this group was 22 years. When compared with the contralateral nonfused side, the subtalar, talonavicular, naviculocuneiform, tarsometatarsal, and first metatarsophalangeal joints all had significantly greater degrees of arthritis. The interpretation of these results is limited, because radiographic studies of the arthritic joints evaluated were not available for most patients at the time the fusions were performed. The authors were not able to show any difference in arthritic changes in the ipsilateral knee when compared with the contralateral side. Functionally, however, there were significant differences between the ipsilateral and contralateral sides in activity limitation, pain, and disability. The long-term functional outcome following ankle arthrodesis was studied by Fuchs and colleagues [53] in 17 patients whose follow-up averaged 23 years. There were significant deficits in Short Form-36 scores when compared with normative values.

The long-term results of arthroscopically aided fusion are available also. Glick and colleagues [54] reported a 97% fusion rate with excellent or good results in 85% of 35 ankles followed for a mean of 7.7 years. Similar results were obtained by Ferkel and Hewitt [55] in their series of 35 patients who were followed for a mean of 6 years.

Recently Smith and Wood [56] demonstrated that uncomplicated ankle arthrodesis can achieve excellent results in patients whose arthritis is associated with a large coronal-plane deformity. Deformity of the small cohort of patients who had valgus arthritis averaged 26°. After fusion all patients in the study had a substantial decrease in pain as well as marked correction of their deformity. Despite generally good long-term results, there are still some lingering issues concerning alterations in gait and adjacent joint arthritis in those who have undergone tibiotalar arthritis.

Joint-sparing surgical treatments

Any surgical procedure that moves the weight-bearing axis medial to the anatomic axis of the leg will relieve pressure on the lateral ankle joint.

Multiple procedures may be appropriate for each patient in whom tibiotalar joint salvage is attempted. As with other complex disorders of the foot and ankle, joint-sparing surgery for valgus ankle arthritis needs to be customized to each patient and may require multiple procedures performed in concert to achieve the desired correction.

Realignment of the ankle and the foot should be undertaken both for symptomatic improvement and for prevention of worsening deformity and arthritis that may develop secondary to deformity. Joint-sparing treatment of valgus ankle arthritis must focus on re-establishing a congruent mortise perpendicular to the axis of the tibia. Without this correction any surgical intervention will eventually fail. Additionally, foot alignment also must be plantigrade or correctible to plantigrade. Malalignment can affect the pressure experienced within the ankle joint. As such, hindfoot, midfoot, or forefoot procedures should be performed as needed in conjunction with re-establishing a congruent mortise. Recently Pagenstert and colleagues [13] demonstrated that realignment surgery using bony, tendon, and ligamentous procedures for patients who had ankle arthritis associated with coronal-plane deformity resulted in statistically significant reductions in pain and ankle range of motion and in improvements in American Orthopaedics Foot and Ankle Society (AOFAS) hindfoot and ankle and Takakura ankle scores.

Calcaneal osteotomy

The medializing calcaneal osteotomy was popularized by Koutsougiannis [57]. This osteotomy has been used as an adjunct to tendon transfers for the treatment of AAFD [58,59]. In translating the calcaneal tuber medially, the distal portion of the weight-bearing axis is medialized also. This change in the absence of other malalignment has been shown to off-load the lateral ankle and subtalar joints biomechanically [50,51].

Davitt and colleagues [50] studied the changes in pressure patterns both in the ankle and within the posterior facet of the subtalar joint in a cadaver model after a standardized 1-cm calcaneal osteotomy. They demonstrated that the center of force as well as the pressure migrated to the side of the talus to which the calcaneus was shifted. The authors concluded that calcaneal osteotomy has only a small effect on pressure distribution within the ankle joint. These findings are in accord with those previously reported by Steffensmeier and colleagues [51]. Although the changes were modest both in terms of location and magnitude of pressure, calcaneal osteotomy may suffice as treatment for mild cases of valgus ankle arthritis and frequently is a useful adjunct to other procedures used for treatment.

Although a medializing calcaneal osteotomy reliably decreases the pressure experienced in the lateral portion of the ankle joint, it may have detrimental effects elsewhere in the joint. Michelson and colleagues [60] demonstrated a statistically significant 76% increase in internal rotation and an increase of 425% in varus alignment at maximal ankle dorsiflexion. They cautioned that use of such osteotomies actually may predispose the patient to ankle arthritis. Clinical outcomes studies looking at the development or progression of arthritis after calcaneal osteotomy are not available this time.

Tibial osteotomies

Most of the reports on use of supramalleolar osteotomy for the treatment of ankle arthritis deal with medial opening wedge procedures for correction of varus ankle deformities [61,62]. There are, however, a few reports on the use of distal tibial medial closing wedge osteotomies for the treatment of valgus ankle arthritis [2,13,38]. These few studies suggest that tibial osteotomies may provide durable pain relief and at least delay the need for arthrodesis. Long-term results for tibial osteotomies used to treat valgus deformity and arthritis are not available, however. The medial closing wedge osteotomy is not difficult to perform, but preplanning taking into account the level of the deformity and the center of rotational alignment is essential for optimal outcome (Fig. 10).

Pearce and colleagues [38] treated a small cohort of patients who had hemophilia with closing wedge supramalleolar osteotomies in an effort to slow the progression of valgus arthritic degenerative changes. Correction of deformity was to within a few degrees of anatomic in all cases. Follow-up, which averaged more than 9 years, resulted in decreased pain, fewer episodes of hemarthrosis, decreased need for factor replacement, and improved radiographic grade.

Stamatis and colleagues [2] used the distal tibial closing wedge osteotomy in seven patients who had valgus deformity at the ankle joint. Three of the seven patients had degenerative changes radiographically. Postoperatively, at a mean of 33.6 months, none of the seven patients had progression of arthritis radiographically. For the group that had valgus deformity, the mean AOFAS Ankle and Hindfoot Scores increased from 60 to 91, and the average Takakura Ankle Score rose from 63 to 86. In the subset of patients who had radiographically proven pre-existing valgus ankle arthritis, these scores improved from 47 to 85 and from 50 to 75, respectively.

A lateral distal tibial opening osteotomy may be used to restore congruity of the ankle joint in type IV deformities. Preoperative cross-sectional imaging is essential to gauge the extent and magnitude of the impaction. This technique may involve creating a fibular door or window to access the full extent of the lateral plafond [1]. Osteoclysis of the plane of the fracture should be performed, followed by reduction of the joint surface to the talar dome that is reduced properly within the mortise (see Fig. 8). Bone grafting and fixation then should be undertaken. The authors are not aware of any publication reporting the results of this technique.

Revision of triple arthrodesis

As mentioned earlier, triple arthrodeses that result in valgus hindfoot positioning place increased strain on the deltoid ligament [7,8]. This

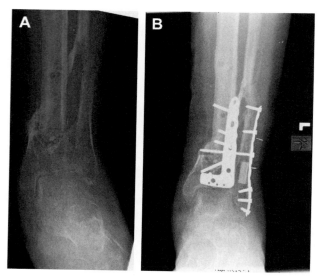

Fig. 10. Medial closing wedge supramalleolar osteotomy for correction of a type I deformity. (A) Anteroposterior view of the ankle and leg of a 27-year-old soldier who underwent bone transport of an open distal tibio-fibular fracture with 5 cm of bone loss after initial stabilization. A non-union and malunion of the docking site with substantial shortening of the fibula ensued. (B) Surgical treatment consisted of a distal tibial closing wedge osteotomy with fibular lengthening and bone grafting. The syndesmosis was fixed with a screw.

condition represents a specialized case of stage IV AAFD and should be corrected early to obviate the need for ankle fusion or arthroplasty. Patients who have malpositioning of the arthrodesis and valgus tibiotalar tilt should undergo revision surgery followed by subsequent reconstruction of the medial ankle ligaments. Reconstruction of a the malpositioned arthrodesis may be accomplished through the use of wedge osteotomies, as previously described [63,64].

Stage IVA adult-acquired flatfoot deformity

In most cases in which tibiotalar-sparing reconstructions are performed, the authors prefer to perform the necessary hind- and midfoot realignments and follow these realignments with ligament reconstructions [26]. Bony procedures may consist of any combination of appropriate osteotomies and arthrodeses, as described previously. Whatever components make up the reconstruction, they must re-establish a stable plantigrade foot and ankle. Attempts to address the ankle pathology with isolated reconstruction of the deltoid ligament without realignment of the foot deformity will result in recurrence. Inadequate correction of coronal-plane deformity ultimately will overstress any ligament reconstruction and result in eventual failure of the construct.

Total ankle arthroplasty

TAA may be the only alternative to ankle fusion if substantial tibiotalar arthritis exists. Because of the preservation of tibiotalar motion possible with TAA, it is believed that this surgical option may prevent or at least lessen the amount of overload, and therefore arthritis, that will occur in neighboring joints. TAA may not be possible, however, in some patients who have excessive coronal deformity [47,65].

Haskell and Mann [47] reported, in a series of 35 patients who had pre-operative coronal-plane deformity of 10° or greater, that correction of joint-line alignment could be maintained in the short term. Despite these findings, patients who have preoperative coronal-plane deformities are 10 times more likely than those without such deformities to develop edge loading of the prosthesis. Edge loading was defined as deviation of 4° or more from the initial postoperative talar alignment.

At present it seems that reasonable results can be expected in patients who have coronal-plane deformities of less than 10°. In patients who have deformity of 15° or greater in the coronal plane, however, TAA incurs a significant risk of early mechanical failure [65]. Long-term results of patients who have undergone TAA in the face of moderate coronal-plane deformities need to be evaluated before recommendations can be made regarding the advisability of such therapy.

Whenever TAA is performed as part of the treatment of valgus ankle arthritis, concomitant deformities proximal and distal to the ankle should be corrected before implantation of the prosthesis. Although some procedures such as medializing calcaneal osteotomy and subtalar fusions can be performed at the time of prosthesis implantation, it has been recommended that more extensive procedures (eg, triple arthrodesis) be done at least 3 months before TAA [66]. Use of an external fixator, lateral translation of the talar component, and implantation of a broad-based talar component decreases the chances of recurrence of deformity when TAA is used.

Sangeorzan's group recently reported that 50% of the stage IV patients treated with triple arthrodeses and TAA developed persistent valgus malalignment [67]. This study was done with a relatively small cohort of patients in whom deltoid reconstructions were not performed. The results of this study call into question the advisability of treating these patients without medial ligamentous reconstruction.

Bluman and Myerson [26] recently described a minimally invasive deltoid ligament reconstruction (MIDLR). Laboratory testing has shown MIDLR to be both anatomically and biomechanically sound [68]. Early clinical results are promising. This method of deltoid ligament reconstruction is modified easily for use with many of the TAAs on the market today (Fig. 11). Clinical studies to assess the durability of correction obtained with the MIDLR will require longer follow-up of the patients undergoing TAA in which it has been used.

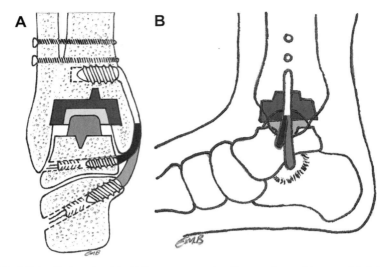

Fig. 11. Minimally invasive deltoid ligament reconstruction may be used to correct deficiency in a patient who has undergone total ankle arthroplasty. (*A*) Posterior-to-anterior view of mid-coronal section of implant. (*B*) Lateral view. The construct depicted is being used with the Agility system (DePuy, Warsaw, Indiana). This reconstruction may be more difficult in total ankle arthroplasties with tibial component stems (*Courtesy of* E. Bluman, MD, Tacoma, WA).

Delayed valgus deformity may develop after implantation of a TAA. To date the most frequently implanted TAA in the United States has been the Agility prosthesis (DePuy, Warsaw, Indiana). The most common mechanism of late failure in the current generation of this prosthesis is talar component subsidence. Although less common, tibial component subsidence may occur, particularly if syndesmotic fusion is not obtained [45]. When a substantial proportion of the tibial tray protrudes beyond the lateral tibial cortex in the face of syndesmotic non-union, valgus subsidence may occur (Fig. 12). This subsidence results from the decreased compressive strength of the bone proximal to the lateral plafond [23] as well as from component-positioning issues. Surgeon adherence to technical considerations will help prevent these problems. On the tibial side, minimization of bone resection, obtaining solid syndesmotic fusion, and ensuring placement of the tibial component against the posterior cortex decreases the risk of subsidence. Patient selection with particular focus on patient weight will help avoid talar component subsidence.

Treatment of the TAA that has developed valgus may be difficult. The implant–host interface should be scrutinized relative to the mechanical axis of the limb to ensure that proper congruent bone cuts have been made on the tibia and the talus. Improper cuts may necessitate removing the component and recutting of the bony surfaces. Bone grafting of the defects may be used also. Similarly tibial or talar subsidence may require

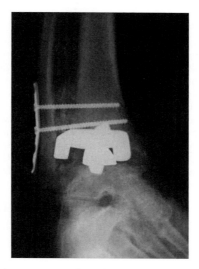

Fig. 12. Lateralized tibial component of total ankle arthroplasty. This malpositioning in conjunction with non-union of the tibiofibular syndesmosis places the patient at risk for developing lateral subsidence of the tibial component and valgus deformity of the prosthetic joint.

revision to re-establish congruent surfaces. Fracture of the medial malleolus intraoperatively may be prevented with the placement of prophylactic Kirschner wires within this structure when distraction is applied, bone cuts are made, and the implants are seated. If the surgeon wants to maintain this fixation postoperatively, screws may be inserted over the provisional Kirschner wires. Insufficiency of the deltoid complex needs to be corrected through repair or reconstruction. Repair of the superficial ligaments is not technically demanding. Isolated superficial ligament laceration will not lead to valgus deformity [69]. If valgus malalignment is seen, reconstruction of both superficial and deep components is required. This reconstruction may be performed after the implant has been placed and will not interfere with the componentry.

Summary

Valgus ankle deformity and arthritis may arise from a variety of different conditions. If the condition is detected and treated early, conservative therapy may provide symptomatic relief and slow the progression of arthritis. Although arthrodesis remains the reference standard for surgical therapy, multiple joint-sparing alternatives to fusion have been described in the literature. Prudent use of one or a combination of these procedures depends on the orthopedic surgeon properly identifying the particular form of valgus arthritis present.

References

[1] Hansen S. Functional reconstruction of the foot and ankle. Philadelphia: Lippincott Williams & Wilkins; 2000.

[2] Stamatis ED, Cooper PS, Myerson MS. Supramalleolar osteotomy for the treatment of distal tibial angular deformities and arthritis of the ankle joint. Foot Ankle Int 2003;24:754–64.

[3] Sarrafian S. Anatomy of the foot and ankle descriptive, topographic, functional. Philadelphia: JB Lippincott Company; 1983.

[4] McKellop HA, Sigholm G, Redfern FC, et al. The effect of simulated fracture-angulations of the tibia on cartilage pressures in the knee joint. J Bone Joint Surg Am 1991;73:1382–91.

[5] Ting AJ, Tarr RR, Sarmiento A, et al. The role of subtalar motion and ankle contact pressure changes from angular deformities of the tibia. Foot Ankle 1987;7:290–9.

[6] Fitzgibbons TC. Valgus tilting of the ankle joint after subtalar (hindfoot) fusion: complication or natural progression of valgus hindfoot deformity? Orthopedics 1996;19: 415–23.

[7] Resnick RB, Jahss MH, Choueka J, et al. Deltoid ligament forces after tibialis posterior tendon rupture: effects of triple arthrodesis and calcaneal displacement osteotomies. Foot Ankle Int 1995;16:14–20.

[8] Song SJ, Lee S, O'Malley MJ, et al. Deltoid ligament strain after correction of acquired flatfoot deformity by triple arthrodesis. Foot Ankle Int 2000;21:573–7.

[9] Merchant TC, Dietz FR. Long-term follow-up after fractures of the tibial and fibular shafts. J Bone Joint Surg Am 1989;71:599–606.

[10] Puno RM, Vaughan JJ, Stetten ML, et al. Long-term effects of tibial angular malunion on the knee and ankle joints. J Orthop Trauma 1991;5:247–54.

[11] Tetsworth K, Paley D. Malalignment and degenerative arthropathy. Orthop Clin North Am 1994;25:367–77.

[12] Mangone PG. Distal tibial osteotomies for the treatment of foot and ankle disorders. Foot Ankle Clin 2001;6:583–97.

[13] Pagenstert GI, Hintermann B, Barg A, et al. Realignment surgery as alternative treatment of varus and valgus ankle osteoarthritis. Clin Orthop Relat Res 2007;462:156–68.

[14] Tarr RR, Resnick CT, Wagner KS, et al. Changes in tibiotalar joint contact areas following experimentally induced tibial angular deformities. Clin Orthop Relat Res 1985;199:72–80.

[15] Salter R, Field P. The effects of continuous compression on living articular cartilage: an experimental investigation. J Bone Joint Surg Am 1960;42:31–49.

[16] Felson DT, Chaisson CE, Hill CL, et al. The association of bone marrow lesions with pain in knee osteoarthritis. Ann Intern Med 2001;134:541–9.

[17] Evans CH, Mazzocchi RA, Nelson DD, et al. Experimental arthritis induced by intraarticular injection of allogenic cartilaginous particles into rabbit knees. Arthritis Rheum 1984;27: 200–7.

[18] Huber MJ, Schmotzer WB, Riebold TW, et al. Fate and effect of autogenous osteochondral fragments implanted in the middle carpal joint of horses. Am J Vet Res 1992;53:1579–88.

[19] Thordarson DB, Motamed S, Hedman T, et al. The effect of fibular malreduction on contact pressures in an ankle fracture malunion model. J Bone Joint Surg Am 1997;79:1809–15.

[20] Lambert KL. The weight-bearing function of the fibula. A strain gauge study. J Bone Joint Surg Am 1971;53:507–13.

[21] Wang Q, Whittle M, et al. Fibula and its ligaments in load transmission and ankle joint stability. Clin Orthop Relat Res 1996;330:261–70.

[22] Mast JW, Teipner WA. A reproducible approach to the internal fixation of adult ankle fractures: rationale, technique, and early results. Orthop Clin North Am 1980;11:661–79.

[23] Aitken GK, Bourne RB, Finlay JB, et al. Indentation stiffness of the cancellous bone in the distal human tibia. Clin Orthop Relat Res 1985;201:264–70.

[24] Yablon IG, Heller FG, Shouse L. The key role of the lateral malleolus in displaced fractures of the ankle. J Bone Joint Surg Am 1977;59:169–73.

[25] Boden SD, Labropoulos PA, McCowin P, et al. Mechanical considerations for the syndesmosis screw. A cadaver study. J Bone Joint Surg Am 1989;71:1548–55.

[26] Bluman EM, Myerson MS. Stage IV posterior tibial tendon rupture viii. Foot Ankle Clin 2007;12:341–62, viii.

[27] Marti RK, Raaymakers EL, Nolte PA. Malunited ankle fractures. The late results of reconstruction. J Bone Joint Surg Br 1990;72:709–13.

[28] Siegel J, Tornetta P III. Extraperiosteal plating of pronation-abduction ankle fractures. J Bone Joint Surg Am 2007;89:276–81.

[29] Limbird RS, Aaron RK. Laterally comminuted fracture-dislocation of the ankle. J Bone Joint Surg Am 1987;69:881–5.

[30] Ovadia DN, Beals RK. Fractures of the tibial plafond. J Bone Joint Surg Am 1986;68: 543–51.

[31] Teeny SM, Wiss DA. Open reduction and internal fixation of tibial plafond fractures. Variables contributing to poor results and complications. Clin Orthop Relat Res 1993; 292:108–17.

[32] Tile M. Fractures of the distal tibial metaphysis involving the ankle joint: the pilon fracture. In: Schatzker J, Tile M, editors. The rationale of operative fracture care. Berlin: Springer-Verlag; 1987. p. 343–69.

[33] Heim U. The pilon tibial fracture: classification, surgical techniques, results. Philadelphia: W.B. Saunders; 1995.

[34] Bluman EM, Title CI, Myerson MS. Posterior tibial tendon rupture: a refined classification system v. Foot Ankle Clin 2007;12:233–49, v.

[35] Raffini L, Manno C. Modern management of haemophilic arthropathy. Br J Haematol 2007; 136:777–87.

[36] Houghton GR, Dickson RA. Lower limb arthrodeses in haemophilia. J Bone Joint Surg Br 1978;60:387–9.

[37] Atkins RM, Henderson NJ, Duthie RB. Joint contractures in the hemophilias. Clin Orthop Relat Res 1987;219:97–106.

[38] Pearce MS, Smith MA, Savidge GF. Supramalleolar tibial osteotomy for haemophilic arthropathy of the ankle. J Bone Joint Surg Br 1994;76:947–50.

[39] Bohm M. Das menschliche bein. Stuttgart (Germany): Ferdinand Enke; 1935.

[40] Dias LS. Valgus deformity of the ankle joint: pathogenesis of fibular shortening. J Pediatr Orthop 1985;5:176–80.

[41] Sass EJ, Gottfried G, Sorem A. Polio's legacy: an oral history. Lanham (MD): University Press of America; 1996.

[42] Makin M. Tibio-fibular relationship in paralysed limbs. J Bone Joint Surg Br 1965;47:500–6.

[43] Noonan KJ, Feinberg JR, Levenda A, et al. Natural history of multiple hereditary osteochondromatosis of the lower extremity and ankle. J Pediatr Orthop 2002;22:120–4.

[44] Jahss MH, Olives R. The foot and ankle in multiple hereditary exostoses. Foot Ankle 1980;1: 128–42.

[45] Conti SF, Wong YS. Complications of total ankle replacement. Clin Orthop Relat Res 2001; 391:105–14.

[46] Myerson MS, Mroczek K. Perioperative complications of total ankle arthroplasty. Foot Ankle Int 2003;24:17–21.

[47] Haskell A, Mann RA. Ankle arthroplasty with preoperative coronal plane deformity: short-term results. Clin Orthop Relat Res 2004;424:98–103.

[48] Lubicky JP, Altiok H. Transphyseal osteotomy of the distal tibia for correction of valgus/varus deformities of the ankle. J Pediatr Orthop 2001;21:80–8.

[49] Havenhill TG, Toolan BC, Draganich LF. Effects of a UCBL orthosis and a calcaneal osteotomy on tibiotalar contact characteristics in a cadaver flatfoot model. Foot Ankle Int 2005;26:607–13.

[50] Davitt JS, Beals TC, Bachus KN. The effects of medial and lateral displacement calcaneal osteotomies on ankle and subtalar joint pressure distribution. Foot Ankle Int 2001;22:885–9.

[51] Steffensmeier SJ, Saltzman CL, Berbaum KS, et al. Effects of medial and lateral displacement calcaneal osteotomies on tibiotalar joint contact stresses. J Orthop Res 1996;14:980–5.
[52] Coester LM, Saltzman CL, Leupold J, et al. Long-term results following ankle arthrodesis for post-traumatic arthritis. J Bone Joint Surg Am 2001;83:219–28.
[53] Fuchs S, Sandmann C, Skwara A, et al. Quality of life 20 years after arthrodesis of the ankle. A study of adjacent joints. J Bone Joint Surg Br 2003;85(7):994–8.
[54] Glick JM, Morgan CD, Myerson MS, et al. Ankle arthrodesis using an arthroscopic method: long-term follow-up of 34 cases. Arthroscopy 1996;12(4):428–34.
[55] Ferkel RD, Hewitt M. Long-term results of arthroscopic ankle arthrodesis. Foot Ankle Int 2005;26:275–80.
[56] Smith R, Wood PL. Arthrodesis of the ankle in the presence of a large deformity in the coronal plane. J Bone Joint Surg Br 2007;89:615–9.
[57] Koutsogiannis E. Treatment of mobile flat foot by displacement osteotomy of the calcaneus. J Bone Joint Surg Br 1971;53:96–100.
[58] Myerson MS, Corrigan J, Thompson F, et al. Tendon transfer combined with calcaneal osteotomy for treatment of posterior tibial tendon insufficiency: a radiological investigation. Foot Ankle Int 1995;16:712–8.
[59] Vora AM, Tien TR, Parks BG, et al. Correction of moderate and severe acquired flexible flatfoot with medializing calcaneal osteotomy and flexor digitorum longus transfer. J Bone Joint Surg Am 2006;88:1726–34.
[60] Michelson JD, Mizel M, Jay P, et al. Effect of medial displacement calcaneal osteotomy on ankle kinematics in a cadaver model. Foot Ankle Int 1998;19:132–6.
[61] Takakura Y, Takaoka T, Tanaka Y, et al. Results of opening-wedge osteotomy for the treatment of a post-traumatic varus deformity of the ankle. J Bone Joint Surg Am 1998;80:213–8.
[62] Takakura Y, Tanaka Y, Kumai T, et al. Low tibial osteotomy for osteoarthritis of the ankle. Results of a new operation in 18 patients. J Bone Joint Surg Br 1995;77:50–4.
[63] Haddad SL, Myerson MS, et al. Clinical and radiographic outcome of revision surgery for failed triple arthrodesis. Foot Ankle Int 1997;18:489–99.
[64] Toolan BC. Revision of failed triple arthrodesis with an opening-closing wedge osteotomy of the midfoot. Foot Ankle Int 2004;25:456–61.
[65] Wood PL, Deakin S. Total ankle replacement. The results in 200 ankles. J Bone Joint Surg Br 2003;85:334–41.
[66] Stamatis ED, Myerson MS. How to avoid specific complications of total ankle replacement. Foot Ankle Clin 2002;7:765–89.
[67] Hall C, Agel J, Hansen S, et al. Complications in the treatment of stage IV adult-acquired flatfoot. In: American Orthopaedic Foot and Ankle 22nd Summer Meeting. LaJolla, CA, July 16, 2006.
[68] Bluman E, Khazen G, Haraguchi N, et al. Minimally invasive deltoid ligament reconstruction: a biomechanical and anatomic analysis. In: American Orthopaedic Foot and Ankle Society 21st Annual Summer Meeting. Boston, MA, July 15, 2005.
[69] Harper MC. Deltoid ligament: an anatomical evaluation of function. Foot Ankle 1987;8: 19–22.

FOOT AND
ANKLE CLINICS

Foot Ankle Clin N Am
13 (2008) 471–484

Distraction Arthroplasty of the Ankle—How Far Can You Stretch the Indications?

Dror Paley, MD, FRCSC*, Bradley M. Lamm, DPM,
Rachana M. Purohit, DPM, Stacy C. Specht, MPA

*International Center for Limb Lengthening, Rubin Institute for Advanced Orthopedics,
Sinai Hospital of Baltimore, 2401 West Belvedere Avenue, Baltimore, MD 21215, USA*

A growing number of patients are developing ankle arthritis from various causes. Many patients are seeking alternative treatment options to arthrodesis or total joint replacement. Most patients prefer to preserve their natural ankle joint and ankle motion. Although research into cartilage regeneration and repair is promising, it is too preliminary to offer a viable clinical option for the ankle at this time.

Joint distraction with external fixation has evolved as an alternative to arthrodesis and/or joint replacement. The technique of joint distraction uses the principle of ligamentotaxis to restore the normal joint space, afford less joint loading, and provide an environment in which the joint cartilage can recover. The first reported joint distractions of the knee and elbow were performed in 1975 and of the ankle in 1978 [1,2]. Aldegheri and colleagues [3], from Verona, Italy, coined the term arthrodiatasis in 1979 to describe joint distraction (arthro [joint], dia [through], and tasis [to stretch out]).

Indications for ankle joint distraction are congruent joint surface, pain, joint mobility, and moderate-to-severe arthritis. The indications may be stretched to include avascular necrosis of the talus. The success of the clinical outcomes varies with respect to the presenting diagnosis.

Existing method and results

Van Roermund and colleagues have written extensively about ankle distraction for treating arthritis of the ankle [4–11]. Their hypothesis for ankle

---

Dr. Paley is a consultant for Smith & Nephew (Memphis, Tennessee), and Orthofix.
* Corresponding author.
E-mail address: dpaley@lifebridgehealth.org (D. Paley).

doi:10.1016/j.fcl.2008.05.001

distraction treatment is that the mechanical stress (weight-bearing forces) on the cartilage is removed to allow for restoration. Weight bearing in the fixator also allows for continued intra-articular intermittent fluid pressure and increased synovial fluid, whereby providing further cartilage restoration. Maintaining the patient within the fixator for 3 months also allows for reduction in the subchondral bone density to increase the resiliency of the joint. These changes will allow the osteoarthritic cartilage to show reparative activity.

The indications cited by van Roermund and colleagues are post-traumatic ankle osteoarthritis with or without equinus contracture in patients who are 20 to 70 years old and have semimobile ankle joints. Their protocol involves application of the two-ring construct Ilizarov device (Smith & Nephew; Memphis, Tennessee) to the tibia with two 1.5 mm Kirschner wires per ring attached by means of four threaded rods to a U-shaped foot ring (closed distally). A talar wire to prevent distraction of the subtalar joint, two crossing calcaneal olive wires, and one medial olive wire through the metatarsals are fixed to the foot ring. Distraction is performed at a rate of 0.5 mm two times per day for 5 days to achieve a total distraction of 5 mm. This distraction is maintained for 3 months, during which full weight bearing is allowed. The device is not hinged.

The authors [4–11] report that 70% of their patients showed significant clinical improvement, including decrease in pain and increase in function (results for 50 patients with 2 to 8 years of follow-up). Joint mobility was sustained with the distraction treatment but was restricted markedly (50% of normal range). Most notable was the timing of the clinical improvement, with only one half of the clinical improvement occurring within the first year after the procedure. A slight increase in joint mobility, significant widening of the joint space, and diminished subchondral sclerosis were observed progressively during the 5 years after the procedure. The authors also performed a prospective controlled study that showed that joint distraction led to a statistically significant better clinical outcome than did arthroscopic débridement of the ankle joint alone [5,7,8]. In summary, van Roermund and colleagues [4] and Marijnissen and colleagues [5] showed that static ankle distraction alone without range-of-motion exercises yields a positive clinical effect in 70% of cases.

Baltimore method

Unlike the Dutch group, the authors prefer to build their ankle distracter with an anatomically located hinge that allows the patient to perform range-of-motion exercises throughout the entire distraction treatment. In addition, the authors combine adjunctive procedures to increase range of motion, eliminate impingement, improve stability, and improve joint orientation. The authors' method of hinged ankle joint distraction, allowing joint range-of-motion exercises during treatment, and the concomitant correction of osseous alignment, muscle/joint contractures, and joint impingement are likely to improve these results.

Baltimore technique

Adjunctive procedures

Blocking osteophyte resection

If dorsiflexion is limited by anterior distal tibial or talar neck osteophytes, the osteophytes should be resected. An anterior incision is made lateral to the tibialis anterior tendon. The tibialis anterior tendon is retracted medially and the neurovascular bundle laterally. The ankle joint is entered through the posterior sheath of the tibialis anterior tendon. The anterior distal tibia then is resected and the neck of the talus deepened. The extent of the resection is checked using fluoroscopy. If plantar flexion is limited by posterior ankle osteophytes, they should be resected through a posterolateral incision (ie, Gallie approach) to gain access to the posterior ankle capsule. To prevent recurrence of these osteophytes, bone wax may be pressed into the cancellous bone. The authors use nonsteroidal anti-inflammatory drugs (NSAIDs) (eg, indomethacin, naproxen) postoperatively to inhibit bone formation for 6 weeks. NSAIDs, however, are not used if an osteotomy is performed concomitantly (Fig. 1) [12].

Equinus contracture release

Equinus contracture can be released by performing either isolated anterior or posterior gastrocnemius recession (Baumann or Strayer respectively), gastrocnemius–soleus recession (ie, modified Vulpius procedure), or Achilles tendon lengthening [13–15]. The authors prefer the isolated gastrocnemius recession or gastrocnemius–soleus recession to maintain triceps surae muscle strength. If lengthening the triceps surae is not enough to correct the equinus, a posterior capsular release might be required to restore the ankle joint motion. Acute correction of equinus contractures should be combined with tarsal tunnel decompression to prevent stretch and acute entrapment [16]. Both the tarsal tunnel decompression and the posterior ankle capsular release can be accomplished through a posteromedial longitudinal incision. The posterior osteophytes also can be resected through a posteromedial incision. When acute release is not sufficient to reduce the equinus, the residual equinus can be corrected using gradual distraction.

Ankle joint realignment

Ankle joint malalignment caused by deformities such as valgus and recurvatum may be the cause of ankle joint degeneration [14]. To increase the longevity of the ankle joint cartilage, reorientation procedures, such as supramalleolar osteotomy, realign the ankle joint plafond. If the tibia–fibula relationship (ankle Shenton Line) is incongruent, an isolated tibial lengthening with or without deformity correction or a fibular shortening or lengthening might be necessary to accurately restore the normal

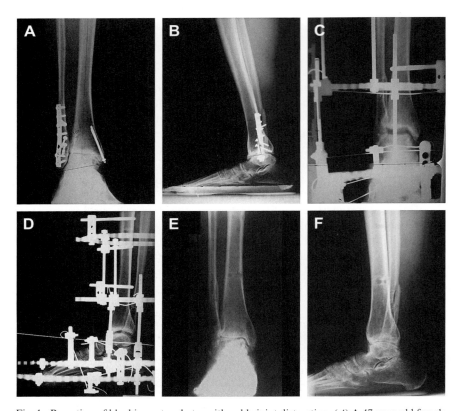

Fig. 1. Resection of blocking osteophytes with ankle joint distraction. (*A*) A 47-year-old female with ankle arthritis after an ankle fracture 3 years ago. (*B*) Note the retained internal fixation and anterior ankle osteophytes. (*C*) Anteroposterior radiograph shows approximately 8 mm of ankle joint distraction. A hinged external fixation ankle joint distraction device has been placed according to Inman's axis of the ankle joint. (*D*) Lateral view radiograph shows symmetric distraction of the ankle joint. (*E*) Anteroposterior view obtained at 3-year follow-up. (*F*) Lateral view radiograph obtained at 3-year follow-up shows the previous resection of anterior ankle osteophytes and a plantigrade foot position.

ankle anatomy. Fixed subtalar joint compensatory contracture, if present, should be addressed at the time of realignment and distraction. Subtalar contractures can be reduced acutely through a release or gradually corrected with the use of an external fixator. It is important to accurately assess compensatory deformities before surgical intervention [14,17]. Correction of ankle alignment usually is done using a supramalleolar osteotomy. This can be performed acutely and fixed internally while the distraction is performed with external fixation (Fig. 2). An alternative is to perform acute or gradual distal tibial realignment and ankle distraction with the same external fixator.

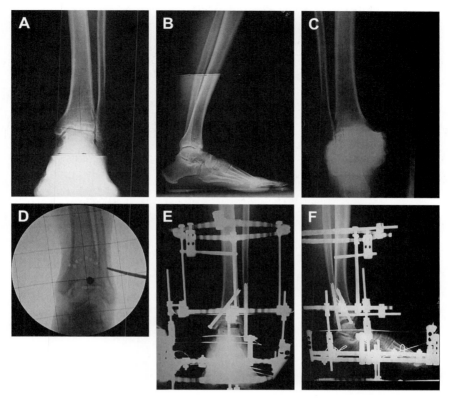

Fig. 2. Supramalleolar osteotomy, resection of blocking osteophytes with ankle joint distraction. (A) 54-year-old male after ankle fracture 12 years ago with ankle varus (10°) deformity of the distal tibia and ankle arthritis. (B) Anterior ankle osteophytes limit dorsiflexion of the ankle joint. No deformity noted in the sagittal plane. (C) The hindfoot alignment view shows the effect of the ankle varus on the hindfoot. (D) Fluoroscopic image shows a multiple drill hole focal dome supramalleolar osteotomy. An osteotome then was used to complete the fibular and tibial osteotomies. (E) Acute valgus correction of the supramalleolar osteotomy was performed and fixed with internal screw fixation. A hinged ankle distraction fixator also was placed. (F) Note the resection of the anterior ankle osteophytes (anterior distal tibial osteophytes were removed and talar neck was deepened) and symmetric ankle joint distraction. The medial ankle hinge is anterior and proximal to the lateral ankle hinge. (G) In the office, an ankle arthrogram is obtained and a growth hormone injection is given at 1 and 2 months after surgery. Three months after surgery, the ankle arthrogram is obtained and the growth hormone injection is given in the operating room during external fixation removal. In total, the patient receives three growth hormone injections. (H) Clinical photograph of maximum ankle plantarflexion. (I) Clinical maximum ankle dorsiflexion photograph. (J) Anteroposterior ankle radiograph 4 years after ankle joint distraction. (K) Lateral view ankle radiograph obtained 4 years after ankle joint distraction. (L) Hindfoot alignment radiograph shows a vertical heel 4 years after supramalleolar osteotomy.

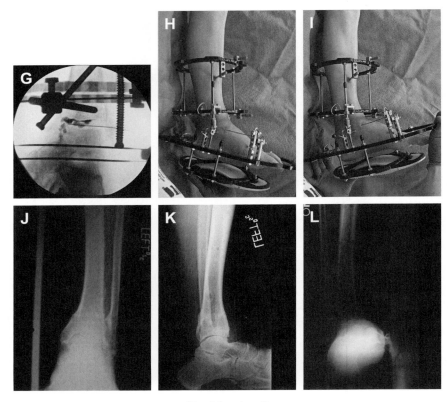

Fig. 2 (*continued*)

Application of hinged external fixation for ankle joint distraction

Step 1

Apply a two-ring fixation block (orthogonal to the tibial axis) to the tibia by using wire(s) and half-pin(s). The tibial external fixation construct should be applied an ample distance proximal to the ankle joint to ensure ease of hinge application. Insert a temporary center-of-rotation wire through the Inman ankle axis of rotation (Fig. 3). Start from the tip of lateral malleolus to the tip of medial malleolus [14]. Then cut this wire short to allow space for hinge adjustment (Fig. 4).

Step 2

Mount a closed U foot ring parallel to the sole of the foot by using two crossed calcaneal wires and two midfoot wires. Then insert two talar smooth wires, one medial to lateral through the talar neck and the other from anteromedial in the neck of the talus to posterolateral to the Achilles tendon. The position of the wires should be monitored with fluoroscopy to make

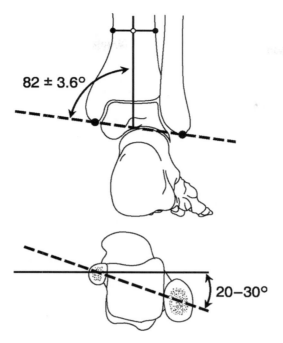

Fig. 3. Inman's ankle joint axis illustrated in multiple planes. (*From* Paley D. Principles of deformity correction. 1st edition. Corrected 3rd printing. Revised edition. Berlin: Springer-Verlag; 2005. p. 572.)

sure they do not enter the subtalar or ankle joints. Mount these two wires to the foot ring and tension them (Fig. 5).

Step 3

Attach medial and lateral threaded rods from the tibial ring to the foot ring, making sure the universal hinges align/intersect the ankle axis wire. The universal hinges joint should be centered with the ankle axis wire (Inman's ankle joint axis). The medial hinge is positioned more proximal and anterior than the lateral hinge (Fig. 6).

Step 4

Add a posterior distraction rod, which can be removed by the patient for ankle range-of-motion exercises (Fig. 7).

The authors prefer to simultaneously distract both the subtalar and ankle joints acutely. This is accomplished by applying distraction between the tibial and foot fixation before inserting the two talar wires. In addition, after insertion of the two talar wires, the ankle is distracted acutely 2 mm and is checked with the use of fluoroscopy to ensure symmetric and accurate ankle distraction. The patient starts distraction at a rate of 1 mm per day on postoperative day 1 for a total of 5 days. The goal is to achieve 8 to 10 mm

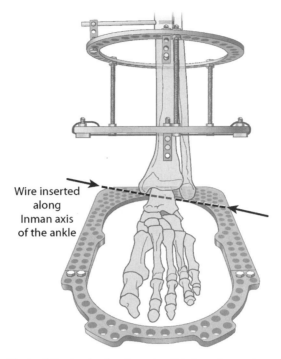

Wire inserted
along
Inman axis
of the ankle

Fig. 4. Two-ring block of fixation is placed on the tibia by using a wire and three half-pins perpendicular to the tibia bisection in both the transverse and sagittal planes. A center-of-rotation wire is placed through the Inman axis of the ankle (tip of medial malleolus to tip of lateral malleolus). This is a reference wire (*dotted line*) that is cut short and used for positioning the medial and lateral ankle hinges.

of symmetric ankle joint distraction. The external fixation device is maintained for 3 months while allowing weight bearing as tolerated. The patient removes the posterior distraction rod to perform daily ankle range-of-motion exercises and attends physical therapy three times a week.

Materials and methods

The authors retrospectively reviewed the charts of 32 patients (32 legs) who underwent hinged ankle distraction with external fixation and who had a minimum 2-year follow-up. All patients were diagnosed with painful ankle arthrosis based on clinical and radiographic evidence, and all patients were told that ankle fusion was an alterative treatment. A total of four surgeons performed this treatment between 1992 and 2006. The following information was obtained from the patients' records: sex, age, follow-up time, method of distraction, length of distraction, concomitant procedures, number and type of complications, surgeon, and preoperative diagnosis. Extensive attempts were made to contact all patients and interview them

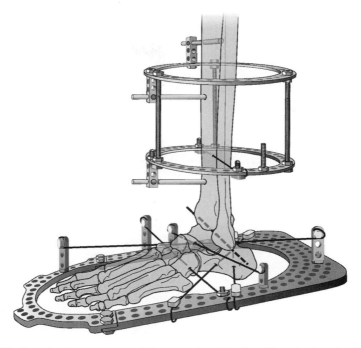

Fig. 5. The foot ring is mounted parallel to the sole of the foot. Note the foot ring is closed/ completed by attaching a half ring to the distal end of the U foot ring. Fixation of the foot ring is achieved with two crossed wires in the calcaneus, two talar neck wires, and one wire across the midfoot.

by telephone or in person. The patients were asked to answer the Foot and Ankle Follow-Up Questionnaire and a questionnaire that was developed at the authors' center.

Retrospective review results

Twenty-three of the 32 patients' charts were available for complete review (9 males, 14 females). Eleven right ankles and 12 left ankles underwent hinged ankle joint distraction. The diagnoses were post-traumatic arthrosis (20 patients), polio (one patient), fibular hemimila (one patient), and achondroplasia (one patient). The average duration of treatment with external fixation was 17 weeks. Adjunctive surgical procedures performed together with hinged ankle joint distraction are described in Box 1.

Complications during distraction treatment included five modifications of the external fixation device, three toe realignment procedures, one incision and drainage of an external fixation pin site, and one incision and drainage of the anterior ankle incision site. Approximately 75% of the patients required at least one course of oral antibiotic treatment during

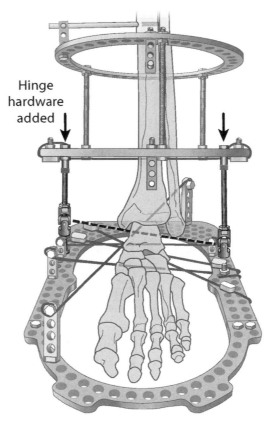

Fig. 6. Universal hinges are placed to intersect the Inman's ankle axis wire. Once aligned, the universal hinges then are mounted to the foot ring. Note the medial hinge is more proximal than the lateral hinge.

the distraction treatment. The total arc of ankle joint motion preoperatively was 28°, compared with the total arc of ankle joint motion postoperatively, which was 27°. Eleven of the 23 patients received a series of three growth hormone injections (10 mg per intra-articular ankle injection) during their ankle distraction treatment. Two of the patients included in this review previously had undergone ankle distraction treatment by the same protocol and opted for a second treatment. One patient had relief for 4 years and another for only 2 years before reattempting distraction.

Questionnaire results

Eighteen patients (7 males, 11 females) responded to the questionnaires. Three patients were found but refused to participate in the study, and

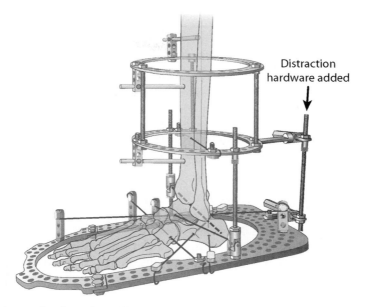

Fig. 7. A posterior distraction rod is placed and can be removed by the patient for ankle range-of-motion exercises. Note the medial hinge is more anterior than the lateral hinge.

11 patients could not be located. The patients had a mean age of 45 years (range, 17–62 years). The mean follow-up period for the questionnaire group was 64 months (range, 24–157 months). The mean Foot and Ankle Questionnaire score was 71 out of a possible 100 points (range, 44 to 98 points). The mean Foot and Ankle Questionnaire shoe comfort score was 47 points, out of a possible 100 points (range, 0 to 100 points). Eleven

---

Box 1. Adjunctive surgical procedures

22 anterior ankle osteophyte resections
Eight supramalleolar osteotomies
Seven lengthenings of the Achilles tendon
Three tarsal tunnel decompressions
Nine core decompressions of the talus/tibia
Six hardware removals
One fasciotomy
One plantar fascial release
One proximal tibial lengthening
Two gradual equinus corrections
Three posterior ankle osteophyte resections
Two hindfoot deformity corrections

of eighteen (61%) patients subjectively reported that they take pain relievers such as NSAIDs occasionally for ankle pain. Seventy-seven percent of patients said they walked for pleasure and 33% said they could run. Only 4 of 18 (22%) patients used an assistive device to walk, and 2 of 18 patients (11%) reported severe limitations. Sixty-one percent (11 of 18 patients) were very satisfied or satisfied by the result of the surgery. When asked about their current ankle pain, 78% (14 of 18 patients) of the patients had only occasional moderate-to-mild pain. Six of 18 patients (33%) reported that they were not satisfied with the outcome; however, 71% said they would recommend this procedure to a friend. Only two patients underwent a subsequent ankle surgery (one ankle fusion and one ankle replacement).

A t-test showed no statistically significant difference between the group with 5 years or less follow-up (n = 9) and the group with greater than 5 years follow-up (n = 9) with respect to the patients' level of pain (P = .187). Patients who had less than 5 years of follow-up, however, had more mild pain, while those with greater than 5 years follow-up had more moderate pain when reporting on the standardized foot and ankle core score (100 = best possible outcome) and the standardized shoe comfort scale (100 = no discomfort). The group with 5 years or less of follow-up had a mean score of 79 points (range, 44 to 98), while the group with more than 5 years of follow-up had a mean score of 52 points (range, 0 to 100).

Discussion

The reason ankle distraction leads to lasting pain relief when treating ankle joint osteoarthritis remains speculative. It is possible that distraction permits cartilage repair to occur in a protected low-pressure environment. Salter and colleagues [18] showed that cartilage repair (fibrocartilage) occurs within a cartilage defect. Fibrocartilage formation is the body's attempt to restore a normal joint surface. Pain from osteoarthritis may be related to the effect of hydrostatic pressure on subchondral bone cyst, whereby the synovial fluid from the joint enters through a cartilage defect (channel) and increases the fluid and thus the pressure within the subchondral bone cyst [11]. Distraction might allow for the formation of fibrocartilage, which adequately seals these channels to the subchondral bone cyst and therefore eliminates the increased fluid (pressure) and the pain. In addition, joint distraction of the hip in cases of Perthes disease has been shown to stimulate epiphyseal cartilage to grow [14].

Radiographs obtained after the external fixation is removed show that the joint distraction space of the ankle is not maintained. This radiographic finding, however, does not seem to impact the clinical result negatively. Cartilage repair (ie, fibrocartilage) has occurred, although it is not enough to increase the radiographic measured joint space after distraction, but merely seal the cartilage cracks and defects.

The authors' results showed that the total arch of ankle joint motion was reduced only slightly by the treatment of hinged ankle distraction. This finding is significant in that the authors' technique of hinged distraction did not create any additional ankle joint stiffness. Most notable is that the arch of ankle joint motion was harnessed into a functional range to the authors' goal of 10° of dorsiflexion and at least 15° of plantar flexion. Therefore, if patients have very little ankle motion preoperatively, it is unlikely to become increased by this procedure.

The patients who underwent hinged ankle joint distraction using the protocol detailed here had promising long-term results. Seventy-eight percent (14 of 18 patients) had only occasional moderate-to-mild pain. The authors' mean Foot and Ankle Follow-Up Questionnaire ankle distraction score of 71 points is comparable to a recent ankle fusion study in which the score was 74 points [19]. Most notably, only one of the authors' patients required conversion to ankle arthroplasty and only one of the authors' patients required an ankle fusion.

As for the longevity of the authors' aforementioned hinged ankle joint distraction treatment protocol, the patient who could be contacted and had the longest follow-up underwent the procedure 13 years ago. That patient still is functioning well with occasional NSAIDs and without further surgery. Five years after distraction treatment, the benefit decreases as shown by the authors' data (Foot and Ankle Follow-Up Questionnaire score was 79 points for the patients who had 5 years or less follow-up and 52 points for patients who had greater than 5 years follow-up). Therefore, the benefit of the distraction treatment decreases after 5 years.

Although 44% of the patients who underwent treatment at the authors' center could not be located or refused to be included in the study, the authors believe the 56% who took the questionnaire were representative of the group. Seventy-nine percent have maintained their ankle range of motion and have no pain to mild pain that can be managed without pain medication or with NSAIDs alone. Only one has required an ankle fusion, and only one has been converted to an ankle joint replacement. The longevity of these results and the higher percent of good or excellent results when compared with other studies [4–7,11] suggest that combining adjunctive procedures and articulation with ankle distraction improves the results of this procedure.

Summary

Ankle joint distraction is a viable alternative to ankle arthrodesis or ankle replacement. A congruent, painful, mobile, and arthritic ankle joint treated with this technique can achieve good results. The à la carte approach (blocking osteophyte resection, muscle/joint contracture release, and osseous ankle realignment procedures) presented in this article is as important for a successful outcome as is the hinged ankle joint distraction technique itself.

Acknowledgments

The authors thank Joy Marlowe, MA, for her excellent illustrations, Alvien Lee, for his photographic expertise, and Amanda Chase, MA, for her expeditious editing. Also, the authors would like to thank Terry-Elinor Reid, BS, for her assistance with data collection and statistical analyses.

References

[1] Volkov MV, Oganesian OV. Restoration of function in the knee and elbow with a hinge distracter apparatus. J Bone Joint Surg Am 1975;57(5):591–600.

[2] Judet R, Judet T. [The use of a hinge distraction apparatus after arthrolysis and arthroplasty]. Rev Chir Orthop Reparatrice Appar Mot 1978;64(5):353–65 [in French].

[3] Aldegheri R, Trivella G, Saleh M. Articulated distraction of the hip: conservative surgery for arthritis in young patients. Clin Orthop Relat Res 1994;301:94–101.

[4] van Roermund PM, Marijnissen AC, Lafeber FP. Joint distraction as an alternative for the treatment of osteoarthritis. Foot Ankle Clin 2002;7(3):515–27.

[5] Marijnissen AC, van Roermund PM, van Melkebeek J, et al. Clinical benefit of joint distraction in the treatment of ankle osteoarthritis. Foot Ankle Clin 2003;8(2):335–46.

[6] van Valburg AA, van Roermund PM, Marijnissen AC, et al. Joint distraction in treatment of osteoarthritis: a two-year follow-up of the ankle. Osteoarthritis Cartilage 1999;7(5):474–9.

[7] Marijnissen AC, van Roermund PM, van Melkebeek J, et al. Clinical benefit of joint distraction in treatment of severe osteoarthritis of the ankle: proof of concept in an open prospective study and in a randomized controlled study. Arthritis Rheum 2002;46(11):2893–902.

[8] Marijnissen AC, Vincken KL, Viergever MA, et al. Ankle images digital analysis (AIDA): digital measurement of joint space width and subchondral sclerosis on standard radiographs. Osteoarthritis Cartilage 2001;9(3):264–72.

[9] Marijnissen AC, van Roermund PM, Verzijl N, et al. Does joint distraction result in actual repair of cartilage in experimentally induced osteoarthritis? Arthritis Rheum 2001;44:S306.

[10] van Roermund PM, Lafeber FP. Joint distraction as treatment for ankle osteoarthritis. Instr Course Lect 1999;48:249–54.

[11] van Valburg AA, van Roermund PM, Lammens J, et al. Can Ilizarov joint distraction delay the need for an arthrodesis of the ankle? A preliminary report. J Bone Joint Surg Br 1995; 77(5):720–5.

[12] Dahners LE, Mullis BH. Effects of nonsteroidal anti-inflammatory drugs on bone formation and soft tissue healing. J Am Acad Orthop Surg 2004;12(3):139–43.

[13] Lamm BM, Paley D, Herzenberg JE. Gastrocnemius soleus recession: a simpler more limited approach. J Am Podiatr Med Assoc 2005;95(1):18–25.

[14] Paley D. Principles of deformity correction. 1st editon. Corr 3rd printing. Revised edition. Berlin: Springer-Verlag; 2005.

[15] Herzenberg JE, Lamm BM, Corwin C, et al. Isolated recession of the gastrocnemius muscle: the Baumann procedure. Foot Ankle Int 2007;28(11):1154–9.

[16] Lamm BM, Paley D, Testani M, et al. Tarsal tunnel decompression in leg lengthening and deformity correction of the foot and ankle. J Foot Ankle Surg 2007;46(3):201–6.

[17] Lamm BM, Paley D. Deformity correction planning for hindfoot, ankle, and lower limb. Clin Podiatr Med Surg 2004;21(3):305–26.

[18] Salter RB, Simmonds DF, Malcolm BW, et al. The biological effect of continuous passive motion on the healing of full-thickness defects in articular cartilage: an experimental investigation in the rabbit. J Bone Joint Surg Am 1980;62(8):1232–51.

[19] Colman AB, Pomeroy GC. Transfibular ankle arthrodesis with rigid internal fixation: an assessment of outcome. Foot Ankle Int 2007;28(3):303–7.

ELSEVIER
SAUNDERS

Foot Ankle Clin N Am
13 (2008) 485–494

FOOT AND
ANKLE CLINICS

Total Ankle Replacement: the Agility LP Prosthesis

Rebecca Cerrato, MD*, Mark S. Myerson, MD

*The Institute for Foot and Ankle Reconstruction at Mercy, 301 St. Paul Place,
Mercy Medical Center, Baltimore, MD 21202, USA*

The original design for the Agility ankle was developed and patented in the late 1970s by Franklin G. Alvine. DePuy Orthopaedics began manufacturing the implant as the Agility Ankle System. Currently in the United States, the Agility is the most widely used ankle prosthesis [1]. With more than 20 years of experience, the Agility Ankle System has the longest follow-up of any fixed-bearing device [2].

Since its introduction, the Agility Ankle System has gone through several design modifications. The Agility LP Total Ankle System was introduced in 2007 as the fourth-generation design of the widely used Agility (DePuy Orthopaedics, Warsaw, Indiana) (Figs. 1 and 2). This newer version features three major improvements to reduce complications: a redesigned broad-based talar component, the ability to mismatch component sizes, and a front-loading polyethylene. This article briefly reviews the history of the Agility Total Ankle System and illustrates each of the modifications made with the LP implant.

Design history

Initially developed for implantation only by its developer, Alvine, the Agility Ankle System became available to a few United States surgeons by 1993 [3]. By 1999, the ankle implant was made widely available to

The Institute for Foot and Ankle Reconstruction at Mercy Medical Center receives corporate support from DePuy Orthopaedics (Warsaw, Indiana) by way of an educational grant.

Dr. Myerson is a paid consultant for DePuy and receives royalties on the Agility Total Ankle Prosthesis (DePuy Orthopaedics, Warsaw, Indiana).

* Corresponding author.

E-mail address: boohinck2@yahoo.com (R. Cerrato).

doi:10.1016/j.fcl.2008.06.002

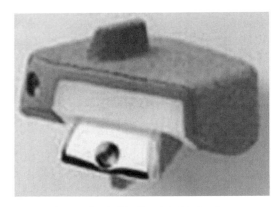

Fig. 1. The Agility Total Ankle Implant.

surgeons who completed a company-sponsored skills course at the American Academy of Orthopaedic Surgeons Learning Center.

The Agility Ankle System is a semiconstrained, two-component ankle design, which takes advantage of the tibiofibular syndesmosis to increase surface area for implant support and bony ingrowth [4–6]. The tibial implant bridges the lateral cortex of the tibia and the medial cortex of the fibula. The articulating surface of the tibia angles 20° externally, conforming to the intermalleolar axis in the normal ankle joint. The implant resurfaces not only the inferior/superior surface of the tibiotalar joint but also the medial and lateral recesses. The talar component was designed to be semiconstrained, allowing mediolateral translation and rotation underneath the polyethylene, to decrease the stress imparted at the prosthesis-bone interface. The talus is wider anteriorly to provide more stability in the stance

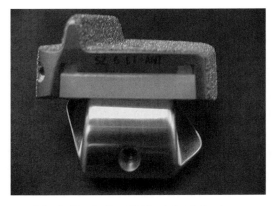

Fig. 2. The Agility LP Total Ankle Implant.

phase of gait. Distraction is performed during implantation of this device not only allowing proper tensioning of the collateral ligaments but also minimizing the amount of bone resected.

The initial implants, tibial and talar components, were constructed with titanium. In phase I, complications, including tibial base plate fractures, resulted and brought about the first modification of the system in 1987. The tibial component was thickened, increasing its strength 400% [7]. At the same time the talus was converted to cobalt chromium in response to the poor wear qualities of titanium against polyethylene. In 1997, the posterior aspect of the tibial component was augmented in phase II. This design change was made to limit posterior tibia subsidence. With phase III, just before the implant system became widely available for implantation, the number of sizes available increased from three to six. Finally in 2001, a revision talar component with a wide rectangular base was made available.

Agility ankle outcomes

With more than 20 years of experience, the Agility implant has provided the longest follow-up studies of any fixed-bearing ankle system [2,8–12]. Pyevich and colleagues [11] reported on the clinical and radiographic results of the first 100 consecutive patients who had Agility arthroplasties performed by Alvine, with an average follow-up of 4.8 years. More than 90% reported satisfaction and the revision rate was 6%. The investigators recognized the influence of a syndesmotic fusion on the outcome of the replacement. Later in 2004, Knecht and colleagues [8] continued with a longitudinal follow-up of the original 100 cases reported by Pyevich and colleagues, with an additional 32 cases. With an average follow-up of 9 years, the revision rate increased by 5% to 11%, and 90% of patients continued to express satisfaction and good pain relief. Radiographic evidence of lucency around the implants was evident in 76% of surviving arthroplasties. They described certain radiographic signs that were troublesome, including migration greater than or equal to 5 mm or 5°, progressive lysis, and circumferential lucency.

Other surgeons have reported their own results with the Agility. Kopp and colleagues [9] retrospectively reviewed the results of 41 consecutive patients who underwent Agility ankle replacements. Average follow-up, including clinical and radiographic evaluation, was 3.7 years. Ninety-seven percent of patients (37 of 38) were satisfied with their surgery and would have the same procedure performed under similar circumstances. Similar to previous studies, a high percentage (85%) of patients demonstrated periprosthetic lucency or lysis mostly over the fibular or medial malleolar margin, which did not correlate with the clinical outcomes. Despite encouraging intermediate and long-term results, the procedure is technically demanding and can be associated with a high complication rate [12–15].

Agility LP Total Ankle System

To upgrade the existing Agility Ankle System, the engineers and surgeons involved with the design modifications aimed to address certain areas that could improve the outcomes and give surgeons more options in primary and revision cases. Three major modifications were created: a broad-based talus component to reduce subsidence, the ability to mismatch components, and a front-loading polyethylene locking mechanism.

Talar subsidence

The Agility implant is a cortical rim support device [16]. Subsidence of the tibial component is not a clinical problem, unless there is a nonunion of the syndesmosis, and a significant portion of the tibial tray rests beyond the lateral margin of the tibia. Talar component subsidence has become the primary mechanism of failure (Fig. 3) [8,12,16]. More specifically, early standard talus components were found to fail because of posterior subsidence. By increasing the surface of the talus, the Agility LP minimizes the stresses on the underlying bone. Conti and Miller [17] performed a finite element study, in which they analyzed the talar stress distribution and related displacement of the component into the talus for each of the four talar designs of the Agility ankle (Figs. 4 and 5). They found that the LP and flanged designs reduced the overall stresses in the talus, in particular, at the posterior edge.

Component mismatch

Unlike its the previous generation, the LP system allows a mismatch of the talar and tibial components, and it is possible to increase the size of the talar component by one size relative to the tibial component. The reason the talus cannot continue to be increased or decreased relative to the tibia has to do with the radius of curvature of the talus. Most of the cases that require a mismatch of the components are associated with a need to increase the coverage of the talus, not the tibia. Rarely in a revision case, an increase in the size of the tibial component is necessary (Figs. 6–9). Upsizing the talus also would be needed, however. As discussed previously, the majority of longer-term failures of the Agility replacement have presented with subsidence of the talar component and, in these cases, the tibial component usually is well fixed with good bone ingrowth into the prosthesis. Under these circumstances, it should not be necessary to have to replace the tibial and talar components. The difficulty lies in adequate removal of the polyethylene liner followed by revision of the talar component to the new LP prosthesis. Because the radii of curvature of the original and the LP talar components are different, it is not possible to use the LP talus and the original tibial component without an interface that supports both components. This is now possible with a mismatch polyethylene and makes these revision

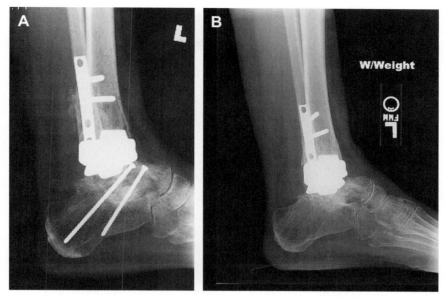

Fig. 3. Lateral radiographs of an Agility arthroplasty (*A*), and the same patient with tibial subsidence after 3 years (*B*).

cases far simpler by focusing on the failed talus and maintaining the well-fixed tibial component in situ.

A question arises when minor talar component subsidence is present but associated with prominent and symptomatic bone overgrowth in the gutters. Should the gutters simply be débrided, or should the original talar routinely be replaced with the LP component? In the short-term, gutter débridement may be sufficient, but the cause of the bone overgrowth to begin with likely is the result of insufficient support of the body of the talus under loads of the smaller talar base plate. Generally, there has been subsidence of the talar component with bone build-up in the medial and lateral recesses (gutters) and, frequently, the tibial component is stable and well aligned. Once a patient is symptomatic, it is likely that the more reliable long-term revision option is to revise the talar component to the LP prosthesis, which improves

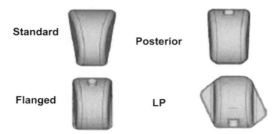

Fig. 4. The four Agility talus designs.

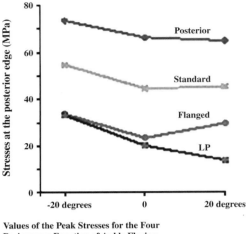

Values of the Peak Stresses for the Four
Designs as a Function of Ankle Flexion.

Fig. 5. The posterior talar stresses of each implant design through ankle flexion.

the surface coverage, preventing subsequent repeat subsidence and bone overgrowth. This is where the mismatch polyethylene becomes important, such that the tibial component if stable can be left unchanged.

Polyethylene locking mechanism

The two-component design of the Agility Ankle System was developed with the polyethylene insert locking into the tibial base plate using medial and

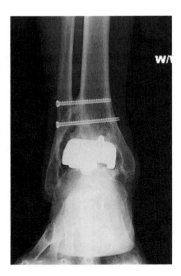

Fig. 6. An anteroposterior radiograph of an Agility arthroplasty with tibial osteolysis and pain.

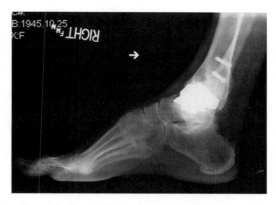

Fig. 7. A lateral radiograph of an Agility arthroplasty with anterior tibial osteolytic cysts.

lateral pegs and a posterior stop [13]. With the need to replace the polyethylene insert, one of the challenges that faced surgeons was trying to remove the polyethylene without removal tibial or talar components. A substantial amount of joint distraction is required to remove the polyethylene liner during a revision procedure without removing the talar component. The Agility LP system now has a front-loading tibial insert locking mechanism (Figs. 10 and 11). This negates the need for joint distraction during polyethylene exchange but mandates that the tibia also is revised to an LP component. This adds to the extent of the surgery and, if at all possible, the talus only should be revised

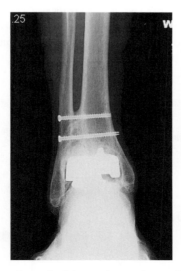

Fig. 8. The anteroposterior radiograph of the previous patient revised to a larger tibial component and LP talus.

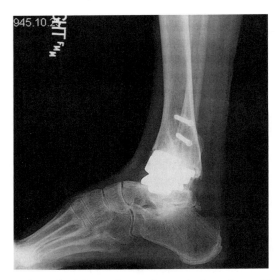

Fig. 9. The lateral radiograph of the previous patient revised to a larger tibial component and LP talus.

to the LP talar component leaving a stable tibial component intact. Generally, the authors prefer to remove the subsided talar component, débride the gutters, and recut the talus if necessary to accommodate the LP talus. Once the LP talus is in position, the foot must be distracted manually to insert the poly liner, which rarely fits under the original slots of the old Agility prosthesis, because there is not sufficient space to distract the joint and then manually insert the poly directly from the inferior aspect of the joint. Because of generalized circumferential soft tissue scarring, neither manual nor mechanical distraction is sufficient to enable the poly to lock in from below. The converse

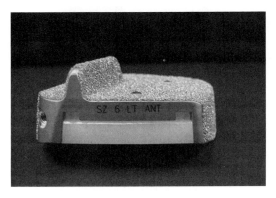

Fig. 10. The LP tibial component with the polyethylene insert.

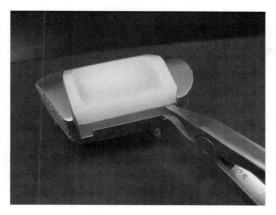

Fig. 11. Disengaging the tibial insert from its shell.

also applies if, for example, it is easy to insert the original poly in a revision case, as there may not be adequate soft tissue tension present. In these cases, in which it is believed prudent to leave in the original tibial component, then a half column poly can be used. This simply is the original poly liner with the inside wings partly cut to half its full length. This allows the poly to slide in under the tibial component without as much distraction. In preparation for inserting a half-column poly, the match of the original tibial component with the LP talar component must be trialed and a half-column poly trial used, which is not standard to the set.

A static test was used to compare the posterior force needed to disassociate the poly insert and talar relationship on the Agility and Agility LP ankle joints when they have a 700-lb axial load compressing the prosthesis (DePuy, Warsaw, Indiana, personal communication). The average Agility disassociated at 168 lb and the average Agility LP disassociated at 179 lb. The sample size for this test was six pieces each. A cyclic test validating the locking mechanism was performed on a six-piece sample under a 700-lb compressive force for 10,000,000 cycles. All six pieces passed the test successfully.

System alterations

The anatomic relationship between the Agility and Agility LP tibial/talar implants is identical. The implant sizing, resection, and joint lines are the same between both systems. The primary implant systems also are biomechanically alike. The revision options to change the joint tensioning are the only conditions that change them biomechanically. The Agility system has a +2 poly and a +2 talar component to alter the joint space. The Agility LP system has a +1 poly and a mismatch poly to alter the joint space. The systems are dimensionally identical except that the LP tibial sidewalls were shortened 2 mm to accommodate the 2-mm LP talar flange. It is this change that makes it critical to use a +2 poly when using an original Agility tibial component with a LP talar component. The +2 poly restores the original Agility joint kinematics.

Summary

The published results involving ankle arthroplasty using the Agility Ankle System are consistently encouraging in patient satisfaction and implant survival. The newest design of this prosthesis, the Agility LP, improves this system with several key improvements. The wider-winged LP talar component covers more surface area and has diminished stressed to the underlying talus. The ability to mismatch tibial/talar components allows surgeons to appropriately size each patient's arthroplasty and ensures maximum bone contact for the implants. Finally, the front-locking polyethylene insert allows for easy exchange of the liner without the need for a large exposure and risk to the tibial/talar components.

References

[1] Rippstein PF. Clinical experiences with three different designs of ankle prostheses. Foot Ankle 2002;7:817–31.

[2] Guyer AJ, Richardson EG. Current concepts review: total ankle arthroplasty. Foot Ankle Int 2008;29(2):256–64.

[3] Saltzman CL, Alvine FG. The Agility total ankle replacement. In: American Academy of Orthopaedic Surgeons, Rosemont (AAOS) instructional course lectures. Rosemont (IL): American Academy of Orthopaedic Surgeons; 2002. p. 129–34.

[4] Alvine FG. Total ankle arthroplasty: new concepts and approaches. Contemp Orthop 1991; 22:397–403.

[5] Gladius L. Biomechanics of and research challenges in uncemented total ankle replacement. Clin Orthop Relat Res 2004;424:89–97.

[6] Hintermann B, Valderrabano V. Total ankle replacement. Foot Ankle 2003;8:375–405.

[7] Alvine FG. The Agility ankle replacement: the good and the bad. Foot Ankle 2002;7:737–53.

[8] Knecht SI, Estin M, Callaghan JJ, et al. The Agility total ankle arthroplasty. Seven to sixteen-year follow-up. J Bone Joint Surg Am 2004;86:1161–71.

[9] Kopp FJ, Patel MM, Deland JT, et al. Total ankle arthroplasty with the Agility prosthesis: clinical and radiographic evaluation. Foot Ankle Int 2006;27(2):97–103.

[10] Myerson MS, Mroczek K. Perioperative complications of total ankle arthroplasty. Foot Ankle Int 2003;24(1):17–21.

[11] Pyevich MT, Saltzman CL, Callaghan JJ, et al. Total ankle arthroplasty: a unique design. Two to twelve-year follow-up. J Bone Joint Surg Am 1998;80:1410–20.

[12] Spirt AA, Assal M, Hansen ST. Complications and failure after total ankle arthroplasty. J Bone Joint Surg Am 2004;86:1172–8.

[13] Gill LH. Challenges in total ankle arthroplasty. Foot Ankle Int 2004;25(4):195–207.

[14] Saltzman CL, Amendola A, Anderson R, et al. Surgeon training and complications of total ankle arthroplasty. Foot Ankle Int 2003;24:514–8.

[15] Raikin SM, Myerson MS. Avoiding and managing complications of the Agility total ankle replacement system. Orthopedics 2006;29(10):931–8.

[16] Conti SF, Wong YS. Complications of total ankle replacement. Foot Ankle 2002;7:791–807.

[17] Conti SF, Miller M. Agility ankle component design: preventing subsidence, a finite element study. Presented at the AOFAS Summer Meeting.

ELSEVIER
SAUNDERS

Foot Ankle Clin N Am
13 (2008) 495–508

Mobile-Bearing Total Ankle Arthroplasty

Alastair Younger, MB, ChB, FRCSC*,
Murray Penner, MD, FRCSC,
Kevin Wing, MD, FRCSC

*Department of Orthopaedics, University of British Columbia, 1144 Burrard Street #560,
Vancouver, V6Z 2A5, Canada*

Total ankle arthroplasty has followed two major design concepts: mobile-bearing and constrained. Mobile-bearing ankle joint replacements also are known as "three-component" replacements, because there are two surfaces with motion between three components (Fig. 1).

Most mobile-bearing ankle replacements have a flat tibial component articulating with the flat superior surface of a polyethylene meniscus, creating an upper bearing surface. The curved inferior surface of the polyethylene component articulates with a matched curved surface of the talus (Fig. 2). Medial and lateral translation at the upper bearing surface allows the polyethylene component to conform to the kinematics of the collateral ligaments, maximizing plantar flexion and dorsiflexion at the lower articulation. Shear loading at the bone prosthesis interface is minimized, creating a mechanically favorable environment for bone in growth.

The US Food and Drug Administration has not approved mobile-bearing designs. Therefore most of the experience and design of these replacements has been in Canada and Europe. Hydroxyapatite coats often used in Europe are not used in the United States.

To date, no clear advantage of two-component versus three-component designs has been determined.

This article focuses primarily on the various design characteristics of the different mobile-bearing designs and reviews the outcome research to date.

Two major forms of failure leading to poor outcome are seen in mobile-bearing ankle replacement: failure of bonding to bone and failure of the polyethylene implant.

---

* Corresponding author.
E-mail address: asyounger@telus.net (A. Younger).

1083-7515/08/$ - see front matter © 2008 Elsevier Inc. All rights reserved.
doi:10.1016/j.fcl.2008.04.005

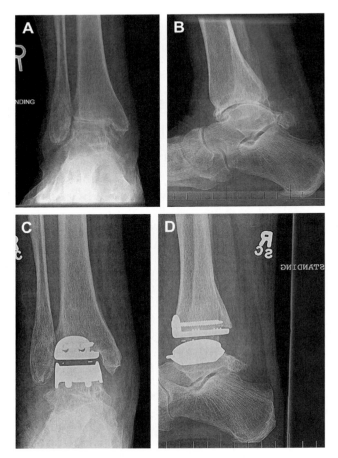

Fig. 1. Preoperative (*A, B*) and postoperative (*C, D*) radiographs of a patient undergoing an Hintegra total ankle arthroplasty.

Currently available mobile-bearing ankle replacements discussed in this article are listed in Table 1.

Approach

All mobile-bearing ankle replacements except the ESKA (ESKA Implants, Lübeck, Germany) use the anterior approach. The ESKA uses a transfibular lateral approach [1].

Distal tibial cut

The distal tibial cut can be made either parallel to the long axis of the tibia or parallel to the ankle joint as advocated by Hintermann [1]. A cut parallel to the ankle joint maintains equal tension on the collateral

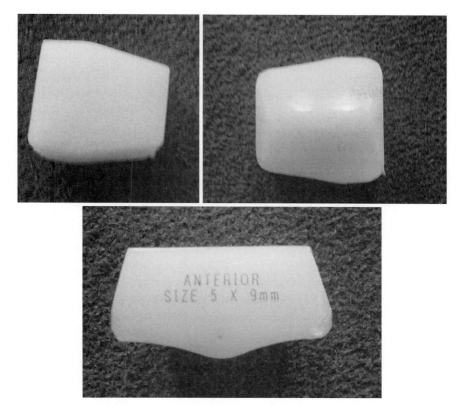

Fig. 2. Three views of an ultra high molecular weight polyethylene insert from a Mobility total ankle arthroplasty demonstrating the flat superior surface and concave inferior surface.

ligaments, but the oblique joint line may create a shear plane. Most replacements therefore are placed perpendicular to the long axis of the tibia, and the ligaments are balanced to match this placement.

Bone–prosthesis interface

All current designs of mobile-bearing ankle joint replacement are designed for cementless fixation. Aseptic loosening secondary to failure of the prosthesis to bond to bone continues to be the major cause of postoperative pain and the most common reason for revision in all ankle designs for which there are reasonable outcome data [2–15]. Failure of bonding of the prosthesis to bone, resulting in pain or likely sequelae such as subsidence or gutter impingement, remains the main reason for poor patient outcomes after total ankle arthroplasty. In the authors' experience the Hintegra (New Deal, France) has the best performance in this regard, although outcome series to date do not support this opinion [16]. Hydroxyapatite coating is

Table 1
Mobile-bearing ankle replacement devices

Name (Abbreviation)	Manufacturer	Location	Composition
Ankle Evolutive System (AES)	Biomet Merck	Dordrecht, The Netherlands	Cobalt chrome and hydroxyapatite
Buechel-Pappas	Endotec Inc.	South Orange, New Jersey, USA	Titanium, porous coat
ESKA	ESKA Implants	Lübeck, Germany	Open pore implant surface
Hintegra	New Deal	Lyon, France	Cobalt chrome, titanium, fluid hydroxyapatite coat
Ramses	Fournitures Hospitalieres	Heimsbrunn, France	—
Salto Talaris	Tornier SA	Saint Ismier, France	—
Scandinavian Total Ankle Replacement (STAR)	Waldemar Link	Hamburg, Germany	Cobalt chrome, titanium, and calcium phosphate
Mobility	Depuy	Leeds, United Kingdom	Cobalt chrome and sintered porocoat

used on a number of joint replacements and may improve the outcome. The optimal in growth surface has yet to be determined.

Initial fixation

Both the tibial and talar components need to be held rigidly in bone to allow bony ingrowth. The anterior tibial cortex is cut to allow prosthesis insertion in all but two designs. For the Scandinavian Total Ankle Replacement (STAR, Waldemar Link, Germany) prosthesis, this stability is achieved by two barrel-shaped fins on the upper surface of the component. The Salto Total Ankle Prosthesis (Tournier SA, France) uses a single barrel. The Buchel-Pappas ankle (Endotec Inc, New Jersey), the Mobility Ankle System (Depuy, United Kingdom), and the Ankle Evolutive System (AES, Biomet Merck, the Netherlands) use a tibial stem requiring a vertical window in the anterior tibial cortex that is grafted to bone at the end of the procedure [1]. The need for a cortical window may cause some initial motion of the component after insertion [10].

Initial motion seen in radiostereometric analysis studies indicates that the initial rigid fixation for total ankle arthroplasty has not been achieved [10,17]. This motion may precipitate fibrous in growth and subsequent failure of the prosthesis.

The Hintegra and Ramses (Fournitures Hopitaliers, France) ankles are placed without disrupting the anterior tibial cortex. Biomechanical studies have shown that the anterior tibial cortex allows significant load transfer [1]. The Hintegra ankle is stabilized by an anterior flange and screw fixation. The Ramses ankle has lugs fixating the replacement by an oblique insertion.

On the tibial side, initial fixation is achieved in most mobile-bearing ankles by the conformity of the prosthesis to the upper surface of the talus (Fig. 3). For the STAR, Hintegra, Mobility, and Buchel-Pappas ankles, three cuts in the coronal plane create stability similar to a femoral component in a total knee arthroplasty. Additional fixation is achieved using pegs (Hintegra), flanges (Buechel-Pappas, Mobility) or screws (Hintegra).

The creation of stable fixation on the talar side requires matching the talar cuts correctly to the prosthesis. Because good visualization, technique, and instrumentation are required, the AES, Salto, and the Ramses devices are implanted using a two-cut technique that involves a greater degree of bone resection.

The ability to match the talar component correctly requires an appropriate number of components, and matching may be better if designated left-ankle and right-ankle components are provided rather than one component being used for all ankles. The Salto and Hintegra ankles are matched to each side, and the STAR and Mobility ankles have bilateral components. The Salto has four talar sizes, the STAR has five, and the Hintegra and Mobility devices have six.

Talar components may have their own cutting blocks or may be matched to a limited number of cuts. For example, the Mobility talar component matches to two cuts, with sizes one to four matching one cut, and sizes five and six matching a larger cut. The Hintegra matches each size to one cut, allowing better preservation of bone stock.

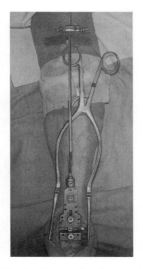

Fig. 3. Hintegra jig placement.

Factors affecting polyethylene wear

One study has shown significantly higher wear rates in the polyethylene of the Buchel-Pappas device than in the Mobility ankle [18]. Fractures also can occur [19]. The authors have seen a number of failures of polyethylene components in STAR ankles (Figs. 4 and 5). Therefore not all polyethylene components are created equal, and the surgeon should know the potential quality of the polyethylene before making a choice of prosthesis. Many factors affect polyethylene quality. A company with arthroplasty experience is more likely to have a consistent polyethylene. Polyethylene comes to the manufacturer either as a resin or as sheet or bar stock created by ram extrusion. The prosthesis company then creates the end product by compression molding resin or by machining bar stock. One study of Miller-Gallante knees (Zimmer, Warsaw, Indiana) found less surface delamination and lower wear in compression-molded components than in components machined from gamma-irradiated bar stock [20]. The benefits of one manufacturing process over another seem to be marginal, however. Therefore both manufacturing techniques are considered appropriate in hip and knee replacement. The method of sterilization and the shelf life seem to be more critical. The surface of the polyethylene and its tolerance to the tibial and talar components depends on the quality of machining. Components should be manufactured from ultra high molecular weight polyethylene (UHMPE) to appropriate International Organization for Standardization (ISO) and American Society for Testing and Materials (ASTM) guidelines. For example, ISO 5834-1 sets standards for UHMPE in powder form, ISO 5834-2 sets standards for molded UHMPE, 5834-3 sets standards for ageing methods, and 5834-4 covers the measurement

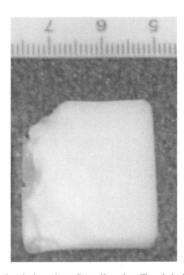

Fig. 4. Failed polyethylene in a Scandinavian Total Ankle Replacement.

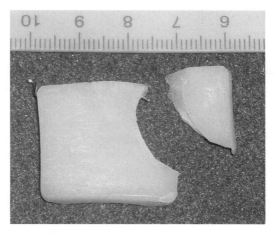

Fig. 5. Failed polyethylene in a Scandinavian Total Ankle Replacement.

of oxidization [21]. ASTM F648 refers to the standards for UHMPE powder and fabricated forms for surgical implants [22]. The component should not be used if these reference standards are not followed.

The material may be surfaced sterilized by ethylene oxide, which, despite being highly toxic, does not interact with the polyethylene surface. Alternatively, the component may be sterilized by gamma irradiation, which may cause oxidation and cleavage planes, particularly if the component is sterilized or stored in air. Components therefore should not be sterilized or stored in air; doing so may therefore affect the product's shelf life. The wear rate in total knee arthroplasty was found to be associated with shelf life, with a 1-year increase in shelf life causing increased wear rates [23]. Surgeons should be aware of the shelf life of the polyethylene components and reject any that are past their shelf life date. Because of the number of manufacturers and variety of manufacturing techniques of mobile-bearing ankles, these factors may be less standardized than in constrained designs.

Once inserted, polyethylene wears by a surface wear, producing particles, and subsurface fatigue. Subsurface wear is higher in components less than 6 mm thick [24].

Different metals may have different degrees of wettability (the metal's ability to support a lubrication layer). Ion-impregnated cobalt chrome may have the best surface characteristics [25]. Therefore wear may be minimized if both components are made of cobalt chrome.

Subsurface fatigue, delamination, and catastrophic failure of the polyethylene component are increased if the polyethylene is less than 6 mm thick at its thinnest point. The quoted thickness of components does not necessarily correspond to the thinnest point [26].

Finally, the manufacturer should supply polyethylene components in various sizes to allow ligament balancing once the metal components have been inserted. For example, the Hintegra implant comes with 5-, 7-, and 9-mm polyethylene inserts. The STAR device has 6-, 7-, 8-, 9-, and 10-mm inserts. The Salto has 8-, 9-,10-, and 11-mm inserts. The referencing for these components may vary, and the authors currently do not know the true minimum thickness provided by each manufacturer.

Polyethylene failure has been reported in the STAR prosthesis, perhaps because of the longer follow-up for this prosthesis [5].

Most designs (STAR, Hintegra, Mobility, Buchel-Pappas, AES) have no constraint between the tibia and the polyethylene insert. In the Salto device the motion of the polyethylene is restricted on one side. The ESKA ankle restricts motion of the polyethylene component in the anteroposterior plane but not in the medial-to-lateral plane. The Ramses ankle restricts motion in the medial-to-lateral plane with ridges on both sides of the talar component but does not restrict anteroposterior motion [27].

Wear debris in contact with surrounding bone

Concern has been raised with the STAR prosthesis because polyethylene can come in contact with the distal tibia. Large wear debris cysts have reported in the distal tibia. No other design has enough long-term follow-up to determine this risk. The amount of wear debris generated also affects the development of wear osteolysis. The Hintegra and Mobility prostheses may cap the distal tibia to prevent wear debris osteolysis.

Tibial component design

In most devices the tibial component is completely flat to allow articulation with the flat superior surface of the polyethylene insert. The component should be thick enough to prevent fracture after implantation. The required thickness depends in part on the strength of the metal used in the component. Component fracture is rare but was seen in some earlier tibial components of the Bechel-Pappas ankle.

The tibial component has some features to allow initial fixation to bone. Ideally the components should be manufactured as left- and right-sided for correct conformity with the distal tibia and should be available in a number of sizes. Many manufactures try to reduce stock, and hence cost, by offering the same prosthesis for both sides. The Hintegra prosthesis has the most variables on the tibial side, with six sizes and left- and right-sided components. The STAR has left- and right-sided components with a smaller range of sizes. The Mobility prosthesis uses the same prosthesis for both sides in six sizes.

Instrumentation

The instrumentation must be of sufficient quality to create the cuts on the tibia and talus reproducibly. The ability to visualize cuts directly and by imaging should allow the surgeon to check the position of cuts before using the saw. The jigs should have minimal motion once they are transfixed to bone. The surgeon should understand the purpose and design of the instrumentation to ensure a reproducible operation. Before undertaking mobile-bearing total ankle arthroplasty, the surgeon should train with an expert or perform a cadaver course [28]. In general the newer prostheses have more sophisticated jigs that allow more reproducible cuts, but the learning curve remains steep [4], and complications are more common when the surgeon is inexperienced [29].

Referencing

"Referencing" refers to the use of anatomic landmarks to ensure that the components are positioned correctly in bone.

Both tibial and talar components should be inserted correctly in all three planes of translation and in all three planes of rotation. The component should not be undersized or oversized.

Tibial referencing

On the tibial side, because the component is a flat plate, there is a fair degree of tolerance for some planes of malalignment. Talar referencing is often off the tibial jig, however (eg, in the Mobility device). Therefore correct alignment is critical at this stage. Varus and valgus orientation of the distal tibial cut is referenced off the tibia for all components except the Hintegra, where the cut is referenced off the joint line. Internal and external rotation is referenced off the tibia. The tibial cut should be made without excessive external rotation or overcutting of the posterior side of the medial malleolus, however, because these errors increase the risk of medial malleolar fracture.

The correct degree of flexion and the extension of the tibial component also are referenced off the tibia. The Mobility device has a 7° posterior slope to the distal tibial cut. This slope allows increased dorsiflexion but may cause an uneven distal tibial cut because of the deflection of the saw off the subchondral bone at the ankle. The proximal end of the stem of the Mobility device also may hit the posterior tibial cortex with this cut, causing a rotational moment arm on the component during loading. Other designs such as the Hintegra and STAR use a 90° distal tibial cut in the anteroposterior plane.

For most designs, it is hard to translate the components excessively posteriorly, but. the size needs to be correct so that the component is supported correctly by the strong anterior and posterior tibial cortexes to prevent subsidence. Therefore it is critical to have an appropriate number of sizes so that the coronal and sagittal dimensions of the component can be matched correctly.

Excessive medial translation of the tibial cut increases the risk of medial malleolar fracture. Excessive lateral translation of the tibial cut may put the cut into the fibula. The medial border of the polyethylene component may overhang the tibial tray, causing edge loading, increased polyethylene wear, and perhaps stressing the tibial tray so that it fractures or subsides.

Excessive superior translation of the tibial cut places the bone cut in weaker bone. Cancellous bone strength decreases rapidly as the cut is made more proximal. A proximal cut also increases the risk of medial malleolar fracture.

Talar referencing

The talar cut for most prostheses is referenced off the tibial side. This referencing can result in difficulties in visualization during cuts, problems in ensuring that the cuts are within bone, and problems with sizing and correctly positioning the prosthesis. Posterior displacement of the STAR prosthesis may restrict the range of plantar flexion [30].

The talar component must be positioned correctly in all three planes of rotation and translation and sized correctly. Undersizing may cause subsidence, and oversizing may cause impingement. Medial lateral translation may be determined off the tibial jig (in the Mobility device) or may be determined after the top cut on the talus has been made (in the Hintegra device). Proximal and distal translation can be varied in most cases by distally translating the talar cutting jig. Options often are available to increase the amount of resection by 2 mm. Anterior and posterior translation is referenced off the anterior tibial cortex in the Hintegra device but can be changed to increase posterior translation, depending on the position of the talar cutting gigs. The Mobility ankle uses a positioning jig to correct for posterior translation to ensure that the component lies under the long axis of the tibia. Once this jig has been positioned, drill holes are made on the talar surface. This positioning then commits the surgeon, via the subsequent cutting jigs to medial and lateral translation, anteroposterior translation, flexion and extension, and internal and external rotation of the talar component.

For the Mobility ankle, the rotation of the talar cuts, the varus and valgus position, and the medial and lateral translation of the talar cut, as well as the anteroposterior positioning of the component, are referenced off the tibia.

For the Hintegra replacement, a similar referencing exists, but there is more ability to vary the rotation, anteroposterior position, and medial and lateral translation after inspection of the initial talar cut.

Bonding to bone

Many of the European ankle replacement designs have an hydroxyapatite coat. This coat may be beneficial in ankle joint replacement. The STAR device used in the United States and Canada has a cobalt chrome ingrowth surface, so results from the United States and Canada may differ from the European reports [31].

Revision components and components for use in primary operations with bone loss

The STAR and Hintegra prostheses have revision components available for use when there is bone loss. Some patients undergoing a primary arthroplasty may have a flat talus, which often is not suitable for some designs of talar cuts. The Hintegra prosthesis comes with a revision component that allows the surgeon to use a flat cut in selected cases. Similarly, the tibial side comes with a thicker component for revision cases. The STAR device has a stemmed revision talar component.

Early complications of mobile-bearing total ankle arthroplasty

Early complications specific to mobile-bearing arthroplasty include a potential risk for malleolar fracture [14,28,32] secondary to the bone cuts resecting bone off the tibial side to make room for the prosthesis. Wound complications are also an issue [14]. These complications become less common with the increasing experience of the surgeon [5].

Factors that may affect outcome of mobile-bearing total ankle arthroplasty

The STAR prosthesis and the Buechel-Pappas replacement seem to have a lower quality of polyethylene than more recent designs [18]. Standards for the quality of polyethylene have been made more rigorous. The authors have observed a higher rate of failure of polyethylene components in the STAR prosthesis than in the other designs inserted in Canada.

Wear debris osteolysis of the distal tibia has been seen with the STAR prosthesis [14].

Failure of bone fixation can cause ongoing discomfort and may require revision. In outcome series to date, there is no prosthesis or bonding surface design that has not had a failure caused by aseptic loosening. The ideal bone–prosthesis interface has not yet been determined.

Outcomes

Three versions of the STAR have been placed: a cemented European version, an uncemented European version, and a United States uncemented version. The failure rates of the three versions may be different. Wood [14,33] reported on 200 hydroxyapatite-coated STAR ankle replacements at a mean follow-up of 46 months. Fourteen patients had evidence of loosening, with eight undergoing revision surgery. Loosening was the most frequent late complication. Nineteen patients suffered a malleolar fracture. Nine had edge loading of the polyethylene, with three undergoing revision.

Shutte [12] reported on 49 replacements in 47 patients. Mean follow-up time was 28 months. They observed failure caused by aseptic loosening in 8.2% of prostheses.

Anderson and colleagues [2] reported on 51 prostheses, with 12 revisions being performed at 3 to 8 years. Seven were revised for loosening, and two were revised because of meniscal fracture.

The designer Kofoed [8] published a series at 9 years follow-up. Cemented and cementless designs were studied in a sequential manner without randomization or blinding. The authors concluded that a cementless design was better, based on revision rates.

The Norwegian joint registry has published a series of STAR arthroplasties. In 212 arthroplasties, survival rates were 89% and 76% at 5 and 10 years, respectively [3]. The arthroplasties were inserted from 1996, and the most recent follow-up was in 2006. Twenty-one ankles were revised; malalignment and aseptic loosening were the commonest reason for revision, at seven each.

In Sweden, 303 STAR prostheses were inserted over 15 years; 71 were revised. Twenty-seven had aseptic loosening, the commonest cause for revision. Polyethylene failure occurred in five ankles [5]. Revision rates were lower for experienced surgeons.

No formal review exists for the North American experience. A Canadian study on STAR will be forthcoming.

For the Hintegra ankle, two studies exist, both by the designing surgeon. Of 122 replacements reviewed, eight were revised at a minimum 1-year follow-up and an average follow-up of 18.9 months [6]. A later view of the same series expanded to 278 replacements showed that 39 were revised at a mean of 36.1 months [16].

For the Ramses ankle, a single review exists on 38 cases performed by the designers. Five patients ended up with an ankle fusion. A minimum of 2 years follow-up was performed. Twenty-eight patients were satisfied. This article was written by the inventors as a level IV study [35].

One article on the Salto total ankle has been published to date. Ninety-three of 98 patients were followed for 35 months. AOFAS scores went from 32.3 to 83.1 points at follow-up. Survivorship was 98% to 94.9% at 68 months [36].

One series exists for Mobility ankles, with revision as the only end point. In Sweden, with 25 replacements performed starting in 2005, no revisions had been performed by 2007.

One series exists for the AES ankle. Of 69 placed since 2002, eight have been revised by 2007.

Choosing a mobile-bearing prosthesis

In choosing a prosthesis, the surgeon should be comfortable about the reproducibility of the cuts and instrumentation. Bone cuts should be minimized. The surgeon should become familiar with the procedure by visiting an expert or undertaking a cadaver course.

Ideally, the distal tibia should not be violated, because doing so increases the risk of wear debris particles penetrating cancellous bone (in the STAR prosthesis) and decreases the strength of the tibial cortex [27].

Immediate stabile fixation should be achieved on both the tibial and talar side.

The polyethylene component should be machined precisely so that the top surface is smooth and the inferior surface closely matches the talar component. Edge loading should be minimized. The curvature on the talar component in the anteroposterior plane of the Mobility ankle reduces strain in the polyethylene during off-center loading compared with the rectangular cross sections seen in the STAR and Hintegra prostheses.

The surface articulating with the polyethylene ideally should be made of cobalt chrome.

The components should bond reliably to bone. Because outcome studies are the only way of determining bonding, and failure of bonding to bone seems to be the main determinant of poor outcome, the surgeon should choose a prosthesis for which some published outcome data are available.

References

[1] Hintermann B. Total ankle athroplasty. New York: SpringerWein; 2005.

[2] Anderson T, Montgomery F, Carlsson A. Uncemented STAR total ankle prostheses. Three to eight-year follow-up of fifty-one consecutive ankles. J Bone Joint Surg Am 2003;85: 1321–9.

[3] Fevang BT, Lie SA, Havelin LI, et al. 257 ankle arthroplasties performed in Norway between 1994 and 2005. Acta Orthop 2007;78:575–83.

[4] Gittins J, Mann RA. The history of the STAR total ankle arthroplasty. Foot Ankle Clin 2002;7:809–16, vii.

[5] Henricson A, Skoog A, Carlsson A. The Swedish ankle arthroplasty register: an analysis of 531 arthroplasties between 1993 and 2005. Acta Orthop 2007;78:569–74.

[6] Hintermann B, Valderrabano V, Dereymaeker G, et al. The HINTEGRA ankle: rationale and short-term results of 122 consecutive ankles. Clin Orthop Relat Res 2004;424:57–68.

[7] Hurowitz EJ, Gould JS, Fleisig GS, et al. Outcome analysis of Agility total ankle replacement with prior adjunctive procedures: two to six year followup. Foot Ankle Int. 2007;28: 308–12.

[8] Kofoed H. Scandinavian Total Ankle Replacement (STAR). Clin Orthop Relat Res 2004; 424:73–9.

[9] Kopp FJ, Patel MM, Deland JT, et al. Total ankle arthroplasty with the agility prosthesis: clinical and radiographic evaluation. Foot Ankle Int 2006;27:97–103.

[10] Nelissen RG, Doets HC, Valstar ER. Early migration of the tibial component of the Buechel-Pappas total ankle prosthesis. Clin Orthop Relat Res 2006;448:146–51.

[11] Pyevich MT, Saltzman CL, Callaghan JJ, et al. Total ankle arthroplasty: a unique design. Two to twelve-year follow-up. J Bone Joint Surg Am 1998;80:1410–20.

[12] Schutte BG, Louwerens JW. Short-term results of our first 49 Scandinavian Total Ankle Replacements (STAR). Foot Ankle Int 2008;29:124–7.

[13] Spirt AA, Assal M, Hansen ST Jr. Complications and failure after total ankle arthroplasty. J Bone Joint Surg Am 2004;86:1172–8.

[14] Wood PL, Deakin S. Total ankle replacement. The results in 200 ankles. J Bone Joint Surg Br 2003;85:334–41.

[15] Wood PLR, Clough TM, Jari S. Clinical comparison of two total ankle replacements. Foot Ankle Int 2000;21:546–50.

[16] Hintermann B, Valderrabano V, Knupp M, et al. The HINTEGRA ankle: short- and mid-term results). Orthopade 2006;35:533–45 [in German].

[17] Carlsson A, Markusson P, Sundberg M. Radiostereometric analysis of the double-coated STAR total ankle prosthesis: a 3–5 year follow-up of 5 cases with rheumatoid arthritis and 5 cases with osteoarthrosis. Acta Orthop 2005;76:573–9.

[18] Bell CJ, Fisher J. Simulation of polyethylene wear in ankle joint prostheses. J Biomed Mater Res B Appl Biomater 2007;81:162–7.

[19] Assal M, Al-Shaikh R, Reiber BH, et al. Fracture of the polyethylene component in an ankle arthroplasty: a case report. Foot Ankle Int 2003;24:901–3.

[20] Berzins A, Jacobs JJ, Berger R, et al. Surface damage in machined ram-extruded and net-shape molded retrieved polyethylene tibial inserts of total knee replacements. J Bone Joint Surg Am 2002;84:1534–40.

[21] Standardization IOf, pp. Available at: http://www.iso.org/iso/home.htm. Accessed 2008.

[22] ASTM: ASTM F648–07e1 Standard Specification for Ultra-High-Molecular-Weight Polyethylene Powder and Fabricated Form for Surgical Implants. Edited. Available at: http://www.astm.org.

[23] Collier MB, Engh CA Jr, McAuley JP, et al. Factors associated with the loss of thickness of polyethylene tibial bearings after knee arthroplasty. J Bone Joint Surg Am 2007;89:1306–14.

[24] Wright T, Rimnac CM. Ultra-high-molecular-weight polyethylene. In: An K-N, Cabanela ME, Cofield RH, et al, editors. Reconstructive surgery of the joints. New York: Churchill Livingstone; 1996. p. 45–53.

[25] Litsky A, Spector M. Biomaterials. In: Simon S, editor. Orthopaedic basic science. Rosemont (IL): AAOS; 1994. p. 447–86.

[26] Chillag KJ, Barth E. An analysis of polyethylene thickness in modular total knee components. Clin Orthop Relat Res 1991;273:261–3.

[27] Hintermann B, Valderrabano V. Total ankle replacement. Foot Ankle Clin 2003;8:375–405.

[28] Murnaghan JM, Warnock DS, Henderson SA. Total ankle replacement. Early experiences with STAR prosthesis. Ulster Med J 2005;74:9–13.

[29] Haskell A, Mann RA. Perioperative complication rate of total ankle replacement is reduced by surgeon experience. Foot Ankle Int 2004;25:283–9.

[30] Tochigi Y, Rudert MJ, Brown TD, et al. The effect of accuracy of implantation on range of movement of the Scandinavian Total Ankle Replacement. J Bone Joint Surg Br 2005;87:736–40.

[31] Easley ME, Vertullo CJ, Urban WC, et al. Total ankle arthroplasty. J Am Acad Orthop Surg 2002;10:157–67.

[32] McGarvey WC, Clanton TO, Lunz D. Malleolar fracture after total ankle arthroplasty: a comparison of two designs. Clin Orthop Relat Res 2004;424:104–10.

[33] Wood PL. Experience with the STAR ankle arthroplasty at Wrightington Hospital, UK. Foot Ankle Clin 2002;7:755–64, vii.

[34] Anderson T, Montgomery F, Carlsson A. Uncemented STAR total ankle prostheses. J Bone Joint Surg Am 2004;86(Suppl 1):103–11.

[35] Mendolia G. The Ramses ankle replacement: design, surgical technique, results. Maitrise Orthopaedique. 61: Available at: http://www.maitrise-orthop.com/corpusmaitri/orthopaedic/mo61_ramses_ankle/ramses_ankle.shtml. Accessed 2008.

[36] Bonnin M, Judet T, Colombier JA, et al. Midterm results of the Salto Total Ankle Prosthesis. Clin Orthop Relat Res 2004;424:6–18.

FOOT AND
ANKLE CLINICS

Foot Ankle Clin N Am
13 (2008) 509–520

Management of Varus or Valgus Ankle Deformity with Ankle Replacement

J. Chris Coetzee, MD[a,b,*]

[a]Department of Orthopedics, University of Minnesota, Minneapolis, MN, USA
[b]Minnesota Sports Medicine and Twin Cities Orthopedics, Minneapolis,
775 Prairie Center Drive, #250, Eden Prairie, MN 55344, USA

Total ankle replacements are becoming mainstream management for ankle arthritis. At most recent count, 23 different ankle replacement systems are in existence worldwide. With the proliferation of ankle designs and the increased understanding of ankle joint replacement outcomes, an increasing number of surgeons have been performing ankle replacements. This trend will create different challenges in the future, the first of which will be to ensure that new surgeons are appropriately trained in performing ankle replacements. It is a difficult procedure with many potential pitfalls, and poorly implanted total ankle replacements lead to early failures and potential discontent with an otherwise good procedure.

Another important trend that is developing is the management of more complex deformities, including varus and valgus, which should never be underestimated. Occasionally varus or valgus is caused by pure bony erosion, but in most cases there is an element of ligamentous imbalance. If the imbalance is not corrected at the time of surgery, the lifespan of the implant is compromised. A simple analogy compares the ankle joint to the tires on a car: if the wheel balance of the vehicle is off, the tires wear out quickly. Even if the tires are replaced, the new ones wear out quickly if the wheel balance is not restored. The same goes for the ankle. If there is uneven wear in the ankle caused by ligamentous instability, replacing the joint without balancing the ligaments leads to early failure.

One of the main challenges in the future will not be whether an ankle replacement is a viable option but whether an ankle replacement is the correct

No funding or financial support was received for the preparation of this manuscript. Dr. Coetzee is, however, a consultant for DePuy (Warsaw, Indiana) on their ankle replacements.

* Minnesota Sports Medicine and Twin Cities Orthopedics, Minneapolis, 775 Prairie Center Drive, #250, Eden Prairie, MN 55344.

E-mail address: jcc@ocpamn.com

option in a specific situation. The goal of this article is to give suggestions on management of varus and valgus ankle deformities.

Leg alignment

The ankle joint always should be examined as part of the entire lower extremity. It is recommended to take full-length standing radiographs of both lower extremities as part of the preoperative evaluation, which is a simple and reliable way to determine any alignment deformities above the ankle joint that could contribute to an apparent ankle deformity. Any deformity in the leg negatively affects the ankle by tilting the ankle joint, which can lead to shear stresses within articular cartilage and changes in contact pressures.

Contact surface area can decrease up to 40% with angular malalignment, which creates increased contact pressures in residual surface contact. Contact pressures are maximized as the level of the deformity gets closer to the ankle joint. Tarr found that distal tibial deformities create the highest contact pressures, with sagittal plane deformities having the greatest effect. A 15° anterior bowing causes a 40% increase in contact pressure, whereas posterior bowing of 15° causes a 42% increase [1,2]. These deformities need to be corrected before addressing the ankle. It is mandatory to reduce the contact pressure on the replaced ankle, and evidence indicates that one might actually delay the need for a replacement by correcting the alignment and reducing the pressure (Fig. 1A–E) [3,4].

Foot alignment

A successful ankle replacement is hard to achieve in the long run without a stable plantigrade foot. It is not uncommon to see a cavo-varus foot in patients who have varus ankle deformities and a plano-valgus foot in patients who have valgus ankles. A careful clinical and radiologic examination helps to ascertain all the elements of the deformity. Specific attention should be given to the muscle balance of the foot. In valgus deformities it is not uncommon to have a chronic posterior tibial tendon dysfunction with secondary foot deformities. In varus ankles, the peroneal tendons might be compromised. Failure to address these issues compromises the long-term result of the ankle replacement. Preoperative radiographs should include weight-bearing foot radiographs. In particular, the lateral ankle view should include the entire foot.

Varus ankles

One should look at the entire leg when determining all factors that contribute to the deformity. There might be a supramalleolar deformity and a hindfoot varus that needs to be corrected. Once all the "extra-articular" deformities are noted, one can concentrate on the ankle joint itself. Not all varus ankles are created equal. The varus deformity could be caused

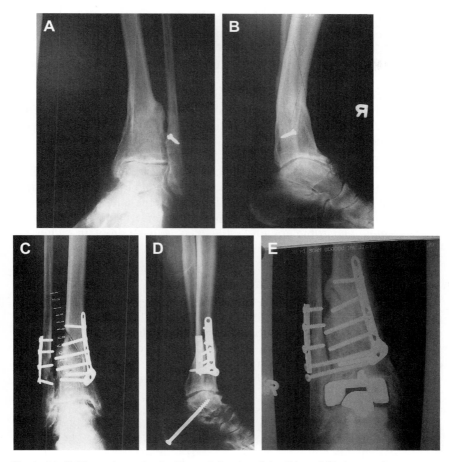

Fig. 1. (A, B) Figure shows the significant deformity of the tibia and fibula secondary to a previous fracture. Significant ankle arthritis is present, probably caused by increased joint pressure with the misalignment. (C, D) Figure shows the biplane osteotomies to correct alignment. (E) An ankle replacement was performed 3 months after the osteotomies. She is currently 9 years out from her replacement.

by bone erosion alone, a combination of bone erosion and lateral instability, or primarily ligamentous instability.

Classification

Frank Alvine, MD, developed a useful classification system for varus ankles and their management in ankle replacements (Frank Alvine, MD, personal communication, 2007). His classification system is as follows:

Stage 1

The ankle varus is essentially caused by medial bony erosion, minimal lateral ligamentous instability, and the following observations on

X-ray evaluation: no ectopic bone medial/lateral, no widening of lateral joint space, or no subluxation of subtalar joint (Fig. 2A).

Stage 2

There is a combination of medial bony erosion and lateral ligament instability and lateral ligament elongation/attenuation, widening of lateral joint line, ectopic bone medially and laterally (especially lateral bone built up along the talus, which prevents reduction of the talus in the mortise), some erosion of medial malleolus, and no subluxation of subtalar joint (Fig. 2B).

Stage 3

Significant medial bony erosion, complete lateral ligament instability, and widening of lateral joint line, ectopic bone medially and laterally (especially lateral bone built up along the talus, which prevents reduction of the talus in the mortise), severe erosion of medial malleolus, and subtalar joint subluxated with hindfoot in valgus are present (Fig. 2C).

Management of varus deformities

Most varus deformities can be corrected, but currently there is no proven, reliable, and reproducible method of maintaining the correction of severe deformities long-term. The specific approach is discussed, but a broad guideline is that most deformities caused by bony erosion alone are usually correctable (stage 1), whereas ligamentous varus or valgus deformities of more than 20° (stage 3) are probably best treated with an ankle fusion.

Deformity correction should be performed from proximal to distal. The first step involves correcting the knee of tibial vara (whether congenital or posttraumatic) of more than 10°, which probably should be addressed before dealing with the ankle joint using corrective osteotomies. This procedure is usually performed as a separate staged procedure. The surgical

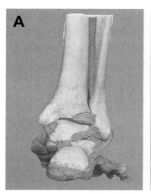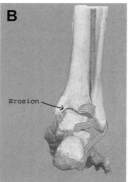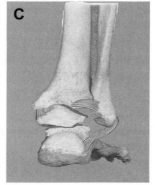

Fig. 2. (*A*) Alvine stage 1 varus deformity (see discussion in text). (*B*) Alvine stage 2 varus deformity. (*C*) Alvine Stage 3 varus deformity. (*Courtesy of* F. Alvine, MD, Sioux Falls, SD.)

approach to the ankle is the same for varus or valgus deformities. The standard midline anterior incision and the interval between the extensor hallucis longus and tibialis anterior are used to expose the ankle. Surgical management depends on the severity and mechanism of the varus deformity and is discussed in line with the Alvine classification.

Alvine stage 1

These are fairly straightforward bone erosion deformities with little, if any, ligamentous laxity. Most cases can be dealt with as with any other primary replacement. The bone cuts resolve the varus bone erosion. The initial distal tibia bone cut should be perpendicular to the long axis of the tibia and not parallel to the joint line. The external cutting guide should be placed with care, and fluoroscopy should be used to ensure the alignment of the cutting block before making the first cut. Because of medial tibial erosion, care should be taken to ensure that the tibial cut is at least at the level of the most proximal part of the erosion, which usually means that little bone is removed from the medial tibial plafond and more bone is removed from the lateral side of the tibia. There should be adequate tensioning on the ligaments to ensure stability of the ankle, which might be more predictable with an ankle replacement system that has several options in polyethylene insert thickness (Fig. 3A, B).

It is important to test the varus valgus stability of the ankle once the trial components are in place. If there is a significant discrepancy in medial/lateral stability, it has to be corrected. Options are discussed in the following section.

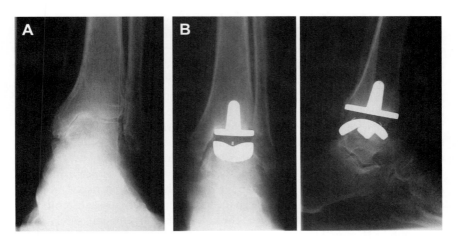

Fig. 3. (*A*) Varus ankle mainly caused by erosion of the medial tibia. (*B*) It was possible to correct the alignment and ligament balance of the ankle with a distal tibia bone cut perpendicular to the long axis of the tibia and tensioning of the ligaments with a larger size polyethylene insert.

Alvine stage 2

A combination of factors usually contributes to the difficulty obtaining initial reduction and correction with varus ankle deformities. The medial malleolus is often eroded, and shortening/contracture of the deltoid ligament, medial capsule, and tibialis posterior tendon sheath is present. On the lateral side there is almost invariably large osteophyte buildup in the gutter, especially involving the lateral side of the talus. Without addressing both gutters, it is impossible to rotate the talus back into the mortise, which is performed using an osteotome to aggressively remove the osteophytes from the lateral talus and medial fibula. If it is still not possible to rotate the talus back in place, one can assume that the medial structures are tight. The deep deltoid is released from the talus by sliding an osteotome or knife down the medial border of the talus until the entire deep portion is released. Great care should be taken so as not to damage the neurovascular structures on the medial side. It is occasionally necessary to release the superficial deltoid by stripping it of the medial malleolus. It is advisable not to release the entire deltoid ligament, however, which may leave the medial complex completely unstable.

An alternative to a deltoid release is a medial malleolar distal sliding osteotomy. This procedure is technically difficult with an Agility ankle replacement because of the nature of the required cut into the medial malleolus. With an ankle replacement in which the medial malleolus is not compromised, the procedure is simpler because more bone is available and fracture of the malleolus is less likely. Distal displacement of the medial malleolus creates a functional lengthening of the deltoid ligament complex without destabilizing the medial stabilizers. Advocates of this procedure feel that as a rule, internal fixation is not necessary, and the period of immobilization after the replacement should be enough to allow the osteotomy to heal.

Once the ankle joint is mobile and passively correctable to neutral in the ankle mortise, the hindfoot alignment is evaluated. If there is a tendency to a varus deformity below the ankle, a lateralizing or lateral closing wedge calcaneal osteotomy should be performed to improve the mechanical axis. This procedure is done through a 5-cm incision along the lateral border of the calcaneus. The sural nerve and peroneal tendons are protected (usually anterior to the incision). A small retractor is placed halfway between the Achilles insertion and subtalar joint and wrapped around the superior border of the calcaneus. A second retractor is placed plantar around the calcaneus. If there is a true calcaneus varus, a lateral closing wedge osteotomy is performed and immobilized with a staple. If the plan is to move the mechanical axis more lateral to protect the lateral ligament repair, a lateralizing calcaneal osteotomy is performed. The maximum distance the calcaneus can translate safely is approximately 10 mm. The lateralizing osteotomy is immobilized with a screw.

Almost invariably a lateral ligament reconstruction is also required to stabilize and balance the ankle. A Brostrom lateral ligament repair is not sufficiently strong to maintain the stability after an ankle replacement. It could be used as an adjunct, but never alone. Several options are available: (1) use of a split or complete peroneus brevis tendon in an anatomic reconstruction, (2) anatomic allograft reconstruction, and (3) nonanatomic repair using allograft or peroneus brevis. The peroneus brevis can be used as a somewhat anatomic repair of the lateral ligament complex. The distal attachment in the fifth metatarsal is kept intact, whereas half of the tendon is harvested as far proximal as possible. In an Agility ankle replacement, the syndesmosis is usually fused with a plate and screws. The tendon is routed around the distal screw and turned down to the talar neck. The ankle is kept in neutral varus/valgus alignment at 90°. With adequate tension on the tendon, the screws are tightened. The stump of the tendon is then anchored to the talar neck under tension. It can be done with either a bone anchor or a small Richard staple (Fig. 4).

None of the other total ankle systems incorporates the syndesmosis in the replacement. The lateral ligament reconstruction can be done in a more conventional fashion. The tendon can be harvested in the same manner, but a 4.5-mm drill hole is made through the distal fibula. The tendon is routed from distal to anterior through the fibula and then turned down and inserted into the talar neck.

My personal preference is to use an allograft tendon, usually semitendinosis. The reasoning is twofold. The peroneus brevis is a natural everter of the foot. By using it to do a lateral ligament repair, you "sacrifice" a secondary stabilizer of the ankle. Even the best peroneal autograft has limited length. With an allograft there is no limit to how the tendon is routed or fixed. A drill hole is made from the "footprint" of the calcaneal attachment of the calcaneo-fibular ligament on the lateral side of the calcaneus in

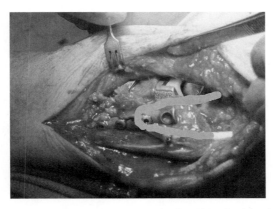

Fig. 4. The peroneus brevis tendon is kept intact at its distal insertion into the fifth metatarsal. It is harvested as far proximal as possible and then routed under the plate, proximal to the distal screw. The screw is tightened while tension is placed on the tendon. The stump of the peroneus brevis is then turned down and inserted into the neck of the talus under tension.

a plantar medial direction. The allograft tendon is then routed from plantar medial to lateral through the calcaneus and anchored with a tenodesis screw on the medial side of the calcaneus. If so desired, a second tenodesis screw could be inserted on the lateral side at the original calcaneo-fibular ligament insertion. A drill hole is then made at the tip of the fibula to exit anterior on the fibula—roughly where the CFL and anterior talo-fibular ligament (ATFL) attachments would have been. The tendon is routed through this drill hole and pulled down to the talar neck. A drill hole is made through the talar neck from the footprint of the talar attachment of the ATFL through the talus to the medial side. With the ankle in neutral in all planes, the tendon is tensioned and a tenodesis screw is inserted on the medial side of the talus. This method allows for long bone tunnels through the talus and calcaneus, easy tensioning and fixation, and reliable reconstruction (Figs. 5 and 6).

The peroneus brevis tendon can be used in a simple, nonanatomic repair. This technique is used in older, low-demand patients or in patients with insufficient tendon length to bring it down to the talar neck. The distal attachment is kept intact, and the tendon is harvested as far proximal as possible. The tendon is then routed under the plate between the two screws for the syndesmosis. With adequate tension on the tendon, screws are tightened. As part of a nonanatomic repair, the stump of the peroneus brevis is routed to the tibia and secured with a Richard staple, which gives added stability and fixation to the tendon transfer. This is a nonanatomic repair that limits inversion but not necessarily anterior drawer stability. If this option is chosen, it is advisable to add a Brostrom repair. The same repair could be done in an ankle replacement other than the Agility replacement by drilling a hole through the fibula (Fig. 7).

Once the ankle ligaments are stable, the foot alignment should be assessed. Any other associated foot deformities should be corrected as either

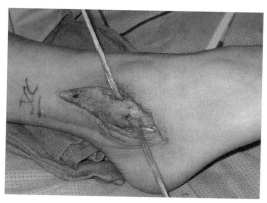

Fig. 5. The allograft tendon is pulled through the drill hole in the fibula. There is adequate tendon length to allow an anatomic repair with through-and-through drill holes in the talus and calcaneus.

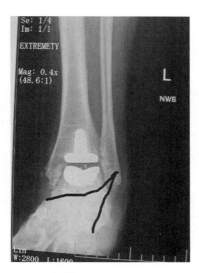

Fig. 6. The shadows of the drill holes and allograft tendon path are outlined.

a staged procedure or concomitantly with the total ankle replacements. If there is forefoot-driven hindfoot varus (plantarflexed first ray), a dorsal closing wedge osteotomy should be done on the first metatarsal. If some of the varus is believed to be caused by an overpull of the peroneus longus, the longus should be lengthened or preferably tenodesed to the brevis to act as a evertor instead of a first ray plantar flexor.

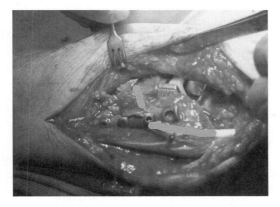

Fig. 7. The peroneus brevis is used in a nonanatomic repair. It is secured under the fibula plate and then brought to the lateral aspect of the tibia, where it is anchored with a Richard staple. In an ankle replacement other than an Agility replacement, a drill hole is made through the fibula and the tendon anchored to the tibia.

Stage 3

The basic premise is the same as for stage 2, but subtalar and midfoot instability also should be addressed. Patients need either a subtalar or triple arthrodesis to correct and stabilize their hindfoot before the ankle replacement and lateral ligament repair. These repairs are at best unpredictable and should not be attempted until the surgeon is completely comfortable with straightforward cases. It might be best to do this as a two-stage procedure. The first stage involves correction of the foot deformity and ligament imbalance. It usually includes a subtalar or triple arthrodesis, forefoot surgery as needed, and lateral ligament reconstruction. Once this stage heals, the ankle replacement is done. If there is significant bone erosion, it might force the issue to do it all as a one-stage procedure. which is a major undertaking and should be well planned. There is definitely a school of thought that severe varus or valgus deformities are better treated with fusion instead of a replacement [5].

Valgus deformities

Most valgus deformities are secondary to chronic posterior tibial tendon dysfunction. Over time, the progressive valgus deformity results in deltoid ligament dysfunction and incompetence (grade IV posterior tibial tendon dysfunction). There are also secondary forefoot deformities, including forefoot supination caused by medial column instability, which can cause or be a result of pes planovalgus. It is as important to correct the foot deformities as it is to deal with the ankle. Without a stable plantigrade foot, the ankle replacement does not work [6].

The general approach is similar to that of a varus ankle. With a valgus ankle there might be medial gutter bone overgrowth that should be removed. A lateral release should be done to allow the talus to reduce in the mortise. A valgus deformity can be more difficult to correct than a varus deformity. There is no local structure (peroneus brevis on the lateral side) with which to reliably replace the deltoid ligament. A primary deltoid repair is never strong enough. If a decent tibialis posterior tendon is left, it could be used as a ligament substitution. It can be left attached distally and under tension anchored into the medial malleolus or distal tibia. This is a nonanatomic repair and has not proved to be reliable (Fig. 8A, B).

Myerson advocated an allograft technique in which he creates a deep and superficial deltoid. It is anchored into the distal tibia, and two grooves are created to attach one arm in the talus and one in the calcaneus (Mark Myerson, MD, personal communication, 2007). Again, it is advisable to correct the foot deformities before ankle replacement. In mild to moderate deformities this could include a medializing calcaneal osteotomy, posterior tibial tendon repair, and augmentation with flexor digitorum longus tendon, gastrocnemius slide, and medial ray stabilization if indicated.

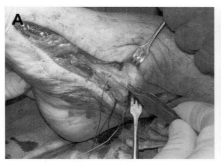
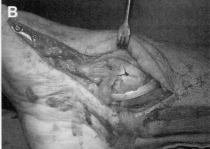

Fig. 8. (*A*) In a chronic posterior tibial tendon dysfunction, the deltoid is often attenuated. It can be repaired and imbricated in a "pants over vest" fashion. As a single procedure, it has limited power. (*B*) If there is still a viable stump of the tibialis posterior tendon left, it could be incorporated into the deltoid repair by moving it medial over the malleolus. It is secured to the distal tibia under tension. A flexor digitorum longus transfer into the navicular should be done to replace the posterior tibial tendon.

In severe deformities a triple arthrodesis might be needed to correct and stabilize the hindfoot as an initial procedure. With the hindfoot reduced under the ankle, the forefoot almost inevitably is in forefoot supination, which is corrected with a plantar flexion fusion through the naviculo-cuneiform or cuneiform first metatarsal joint. With the foot stabilized, the deltoid is tested. If there is an obvious instability, the deltoid ligament should be repaired/reconstructed at this point. The patient should be immobilized for at least 6 weeks to allow everything to heal. I believe one should re-examine the ankle at 3 to 6 months before going ahead with an ankle replacement. If the ankle seems to be stable, an ankle replacement could be attempted. If the deltoid reconstruction failed even with the foot reconstruction, an ankle replacement is not indicated and fusion should be considered (Fig. 9A, B).

Summary

Ankle replacement surgery could be a valuable option in treating ankle arthritis. Great care should be taken, however, to choose appropriate patients for the procedure. Potential complications after failed total ankle replacement could be harder to solve than failed fusions. Although it is technically possible, it is not advisable to replace ankles with significant medial or lateral instability. The complication rate, especially the early failure rate, is unacceptably high. After discussing my personal results with many other surgeons who have performed more than 200 ankle replacements, I believe the arbitrary cut-off is 15° of varus or valgus ligamentous instability. Twenty degrees should be a hard cut-off point. Tilting caused by bony erosion is not as important. Most, if not all, of the bony deformity is corrected with the bone cuts. Failure to correct ankle, hindfoot, and forefoot alignment before completing total ankle replacement or ensuring adequate

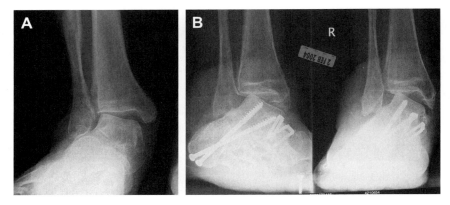

Fig. 9. (*A*) The significant dorsolateral peritalar subluxation is noted in this longstanding posterior tibial tendon dysfunction. The deltoid also appears unstable. A two-staged procedure was planned, first to do a triple arthrodesis to correct the foot deformity and hindfoot valgus, gastrocnemius lengthening, and deltoid repair. (*B*) The patient returned after 4 months for radiographs before ankle replacement. It is obvious that the Deltoid repair failed even with the foot alignment and mechanical axis corrected. This patient is not a candidate for an ankle replacement.

correction and stability before performing total ankle replacement leads to premature failure and suboptimal results.

References

[1] Coetzee JC, Castro MD. Accurate measurement of ankle range of motion after total ankle arthroplasty. Clin Orthop Relat Res 2004;(424):27–31.

[2] Tarr RR, Resnick CT, Wagner KS, et al. Changes in tibiotalar joint contact areas following experimentally induced tibial angular deformities. Clin Orthop Relat Res 1985;(199):72–80.

[3] Stamatis ED, Cooper PS, Myerson MS. Supramalleolar osteotomy for the treatment of distal tibial angular deformities and arthritis of the ankle. Foot Ankle Int 2003;24(10):754–64.

[4] Pagenstert GI, Hintermann B, Barg A, et al. Realignment surgery as alternative treatment of varus and valgus ankle osteoarthritis. Clin Orthop Relat Res 2007;462:156–68.

[5] Smith R, Wood PL. Arthrodesis of the ankle in the presence of a large deformity in the coronal plane. J Bone Joint Surg Br 2007;89(5):615–9.

[6] Gibson V, Prieskorn D. The valgus ankle. Foot Ankle Clin 2007;12(1):15–27.

ELSEVIER
SAUNDERS

Foot Ankle Clin N Am
13 (2008) 521–538

FOOT AND
ANKLE CLINICS

Primary and Revision Total Ankle Replacement Using Custom-Designed Prostheses

Mark S. Myerson, MD*, Hugh Y. Won, MBBS

Institute for Foot and Ankle Reconstruction, Mercy Medical Center, 301 St. Paul Place, Baltimore, MD 21202, USA

Over the past decade, a resurgence of interest in total ankle replacements has occurred, largely because of an improved understanding of ankle kinematics, better implant designs, and advances in surgical techniques that produce better results and long-term outcomes. As a result, current implants have experienced greater popularity. However, the longevity of these arthroplasties, regardless of design, has, as yet, an unpredictable long-term survivorship. Apart from the short-term failures, which are mostly related to wound healing, it is the longer-term potential for complications that is of greater concern. If one considers the potential for failure of a primary joint replacement because of poor bone quality (either as a result of osteopenia or avascular necrosis) and the intermediate and longer term complications like osteolysis, subsidence, and loosening, then one has to consider carefully the available salvage options.

Conversion to arthrodesis in the setting of significant bone loss is complicated; it is associated with a high rate of nonunion and the associated problems of stiffness and progressive degeneration of the adjacent joints of the hindfoot and transverse tarsal joints. The inherent problem with salvage is the loss of structural bone support resulting from osteolysis or subsidence, such that an in situ arthrodesis is invariably not possible. A large structural bone block arthrodesis is generally needed, and frequently has to include the ankle and subtalar joints to ensure rigid fixation and solid fusion. This

The Institute for Foot and Ankle Reconstruction at Mercy Medical Center receives corporate support from DePuy (Warsaw, Indiana) by way of an educational grant.

Dr. Myerson is a paid consultant for DePuy and receives royalties on the Agility Total Ankle Prosthesis (DePuy Orthopaedics, Warsaw, Indiana).

* Corresponding author.

E-mail address: mark4feet@aol.com (M.S. Myerson).

doi:10.1016/j.fcl.2008.05.005

tibiotalocalcaneal (or, if the bone loss is more severe, a tibiocalcaneal arthrodesis) is obviously not as functional or physiologic as a mobile ankle joint. However, despite the difficulties, bone block arthrodesis must remain an option when gross massive bone loss, severe osteopenia, compromised skin, recent infection, or unreconstructable deformity occur.

In the revision setting, a standard (noncustom) prosthesis is often not feasible if extensive osteolysis or a sizeable bone defect is present. Not all revision arthroplasty procedures require a custom prosthesis because many can be satisfactorily revised with a different type of prosthesis (ie, a different manufacturer), larger components, or either of these in combination with bone graft. Where bone is structurally compromised, a custom talar or tibial long-stemmed implant with the correct angle, length, and thickness of the base plate can provide immediate and stable fixation. These special designs now make it possible to reconstruct many previously unsalvageable failed ankle replacements. Arthrodesis should therefore no longer be the default end point. However, the indications for the use of a custom prosthesis may not be limited to complex revision procedures; it may be useful for difficult primary ankle joint replacements where bone quality and anatomy is compromised and initial component stability or support is not readily achievable with standard components.

In this article, the authors discuss the history and problems of total ankle replacement failures, and the indications and rationale for revision, the surgical technique, and tips and pitfalls for using custom replacement prosthesis.

Failure of total ankle replacements

Historically, total ankle replacements have come into and out of fashion, as enthusiastic surgeons took on the procedure expecting success similar to that of total joint replacements of the hips and knees. Unfortunately, the results of the earlier generation of total ankle systems were disappointing, and all these designs were eventually abandoned. During the 1980s, ankle arthroplasty fell out of favor and the pendulum moved in the direction of a more predictable procedure, such as ankle arthrodesis. However, ankle arthrodesis, too, was associated with various short- and long-term disadvantages, in particular, the rather predictable development of adjacent joints arthritis. With an increased understanding of the kinematics of the ankle, improved implant design, and more precise indications and contraindications for ankle replacement, the newer generation designs have become popular as a credible and successful treatment option in appropriately selected patients. Recent literature reviews have presented comparable results between ankle replacements and arthrodesis [1].

Failure of ankle replacements occurs because of patient, implant, or surgical factors, or a combination thereof. Poor selection of patients because of physiologic (comorbidities, obesity), psychologic, and lifestyle (occupational and recreational) factors can jeopardize the outcome. Outcomes can be affected by surgical decisions or techniques affecting implant choice, sizing, placement and alignment, by balancing of varus and valgus deformity, and by adequately addressing coexisting hindfoot arthritis and deformities. Other uncontrollable factors, such as soft tissue complications, wound breakdown, deep infections, intraoperative technical failures, and fractures of bone or components, can also cause failure.

Later failures are usually mechanical, and have been the subject of much research [2]. Similar to the experiences of total hip and knee replacements, osteolysis and loosening, whether stimulated by polyethylene wear particles, or as a result of deep infection, present difficult challenges for treatment. With loosening and subsidence of the components, joint mechanics are disrupted and particle generation is accelerated, perpetuating the problem cycle. Talar component subsidence is considered the primary mechanism of failure of some total ankle system designs [3]. Less often, the tibial component can also collapse into the tibia, as has been noted for the Agility ankle replacement together with failure of syndesmosis arthrodesis [2]. Other predisposing factors include osteopenia, obesity, or overload from excessive activity, which lead to subsidence of either component. Structural weakening of the bone support as a result of initial bone overresection, osteolysis, aseptic loosening, or previous infection will compound these problems.

These structural abnormalities do not preclude revision with a standard prosthesis. Fig. 1 is an intraoperative photograph of a patient who had severe osteolysis as a result of polyethylene wear microparticles. Despite the defect, cortical bone support was adequate to allow treatment with a standard primary prosthesis and extensive cancellous bone grafting.

Many first-generation implants were cemented and, although this could provide early component stability, the static interface deteriorated with time. These implants were therefore ultimately prone to loosening, subsequent osteolysis, subsidence, and mechanical failure (Fig. 2). Resecting

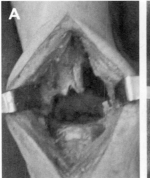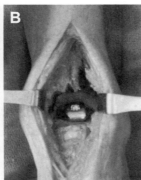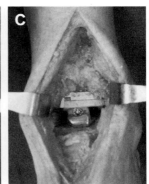

Fig. 1. (*A*) Note the extensive cystic bone defects in this intraoperative photograph 5 years following primary ankle replacement. (*B*, *C*) A standard Agility LP ankle prosthesis was implanted with extensive cancellous bone grafting to support the tibial component.

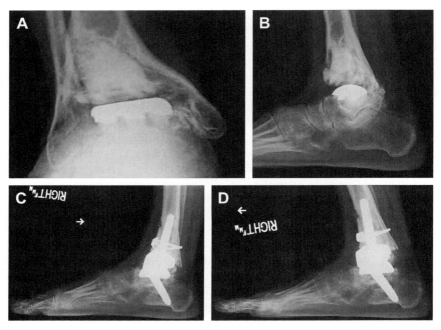

Fig. 2. (*A*, *B*) Preoperative radiographs of a huge tibial defect as a result of the bone cement mantle and cystic bone lysis 21 years after this ankle replacement. (*C*, *D*) Postoperative range-of-motion radiographs 3 years after the revision replacement using a long-stemmed tibial and talar component. Distally, a plate was used to secure the anterior tibial access window for the long stem. The tibial window always heals and should not be a concern.

more of the subchondral bone to accommodate the cement also placed the load on structurally weaker metaphyseal bone. These failures were almost impossible to salvage with a standard prosthesis, and a custom device that could be templated and sized according to the defect of the tibia and or the talus was ideal.

Second-generation total ankle implant systems have overcome the problem of cement interface bone lysis by using more conservative bone cuts and engaging a biologic interface with porous coating to allow bony ingrowth. Hydroxyapatite is also added in some newer implants. To reduce subsidence, many systems have increased the surface area of the components to decrease local contact pressure. In addition to having a wider "footprint" surface for the talar component to maximize cortical rim support, the Agility LP ankle system (DePuy, Warsaw, Indiana) is unique in also incorporating fusion of the distal tibiofibular syndesmosis [4], which provides an increased platform for the tibial component, with load-sharing by the fibula. However, if nonunion of the syndesmosis occurs, this characteristic can become a weakness of this system, causing "mechanical" lysis from persistent micromotion [2].

The early detection of loosening and subsidence is not easy, requiring a high index of suspicion, a thorough history and examination, and various investigations to confirm the type of loosening. Particularly on the talar component side, many designs are difficult to evaluate radiologically because one cannot see if any structural loss of bone support exists underneath. For example, in the STAR and Hintegra systems, the talar component covers the body of the talus, which can "hide" what is going on underneath it, masking bone necrosis. Component migration of more than 5 mm or more than 5° [2] is regarded as the level corresponding to implant instability and loosening. Earlier signs, such as periprosthetic radiolucent lines, should also be noted on serial follow-up radiographs. CT scans are helpful in evaluating for cystic defects or loosening, as are blood tests to help rule out infection.

The improved understanding of ankle kinematics has also been critical in reducing polyethylene wear. Earlier designs assumed that the ankle functioned as a simple hinge, and by using fixed-bearing and highly constrained congruent surfaces, they placed high stresses on the implant articulation and the bone–implant interfaces. These factors may have contributed to accelerated wear, implant breakage, and loosening. Newer implants have improved kinematics, being fixed bearing and semiconstrained, or using mobile-bearing designs to allow for natural translation and rotation. Using newer-generation, cross-linked ultra-high molecular weight polyethylene with improved mechanical properties should also reduce wear particles generation.

Diagnosis and patient evaluation

"Expansile" osteolysis due to polyethylene wear debris tends to progress and may destabilize the implant, leading to loosening and possible periprosthetic fractures. Timely revision may be required to prevent catastrophic mechanical failure and to preserve and supplement the remaining bone support. These failures tend to appear from 3 years postoperative onwards, and are more likely to progress if on the talar side. No studies exist that quantify the rate and exact likelihood of bone defect progression. The clinical problem and therapeutic dilemma here is what to do if a patient is asymptomatic, having good range of motion and an apparently stable prosthesis on radiographs and CT but large osteolytic cysts. Timely revision may be required, but it is hard to convince a patient to undergo a revision when he or she is entirely asymptomatic. Serial investigations and close follow-up examination are recommended to help make the decision with the patient as to when to perform a revision or bone grafting.

For the symptomatic patient, before primary or revision replacement, the surgeon must take various factors into consideration. Although we may have the technical ability and the wherewithal to perform a joint replacement, the question to ask first is whether the patient would be better off with an arthrodesis. Some patients have poor bone quality, and for these patients, an arthrodesis may be a better choice. To some extent, one has to be careful not to introduce personal surgeon bias into the decision-making process. Surgeons have a tendency to favor their preferred procedure without adequate patient evaluation and counseling. This issue is particularly important with these patients, who have potentially already undergone devastating prosthesis failure, only to deal with another prolonged surgical recovery. A complex bone block tibiotalocalcaneal or tibiocalcaneal arthrodesis may not be for every surgeon to attempt, and this, too, applies to use of the custom ankle prosthesis.

Despite the reported similarity in outcomes of primary ankle joint replacement in patients who have and do not have rheumatoid arthritis [5–7], osteopenia and, in particular, avascular necrosis may still be a contraindication to standard ankle replacement. A patient who is more active, is in an occupation that is more labor intensive, or is overweight may also not be an ideal candidate for a standard prosthesis. A custom prosthesis, in particular a custom long-stemmed talus, may be ideal as a primary joint replacement. Frequently, patients are told that "nothing more can be done," leaving arthrodesis the only option. This assumption may be correct, but it requires careful counseling of the patient because a large bone block arthrodesis may be frustratingly difficult and involve a protracted recovery. In comparison, a press-fit custom prosthesis may enable the patient to commence bearing of weight and rehabilitation promptly, once the incision has healed.

A custom prosthesis may also be indicated in a patient who is obese. Although larger standard prostheses are available, these prostheses depend on the proportionate size of the ankle relative to the patient. One problem that we face is the obese shorter patient who has a small ankle or small bony anatomy. For this reason, the authors use a body mass index of less than 35 as the cutoff for a standard ankle replacement and, if the patient meets other criteria for replacement, a custom prosthesis is considered.

The most common indication for a custom prosthesis is the failed ankle replacement, particularly when mechanical failure resulting from severe osteolysis, loosening, and subsidence takes place. The loss of bone, usually in the remaining talus, can make revision too difficult with a standard implant because supportive bone is insufficient, making it difficult to achieve stability and fixation with a standard component. With talar subsidence, for instance, the supportive talar body is crushed and the component is pushed inferiorly into the talus. The previous supportive rim of cortical bone also becomes the source of impingement, limiting range of motion. The overhanging bone in the medial and lateral gutter can be debrided and decompressed; however, the structurally compromised base is vulnerable to further subsidence and eventual fracture of the remaining talus. Although this debridement, performed as either an open or an arthroscopic procedure, can be considered, in the long-term it may not be mechanically sound simply

to decompress the impinging bone. Although revision of the talar component, bone grafting, and use of a standard component may be possible,
the same loads are present and failure may recur. A long-stemmed custom
implant would transfer the load to the calcaneus, providing stability during
the bone graft incorporation and while implant interface bony ingrowth
occurs. Loss of bone may also occur through infection. Provided the bone
loss is not too significant and the infection has been eradicated, a custom
prosthesis revision may be satisfactorily performed (Fig. 3).

A custom prosthesis is not necessary for all these revision cases. At times,
a larger type of prosthesis, such as the Agility LP (DePuy, Warsaw, Indiana)
can be considered, because the size of this prosthesis is larger than other
commonly used prostheses and may adequately "fill" any bone void, particularly in the tibia. Revisions using standard primary components can still be
successful for management of contained defects, which can be bone grafted,
and smaller central segmental deficiencies can be supported with structural
graft. As an alternative to structural or cancellous bone graft, bone cement
can sometimes be used, adding to early stability, for example, at the keel section of the tibial component to restrict rotational and translational motion.

The custom prosthesis

The Agility custom prosthesis system has been a successful treatment
solution for difficult primary and revision ankle arthroplasty cases. The
stems of the talar and tibial components can be fabricated to the required
angle, diameter, and length relative to the calcaneus. The body section
can also be enhanced to the desired thickness and inclination, to act as augmentation for the anticipated bone loss or defects of the talus and the subtalar joint (Figs. 4–8). In addition to the flat, supportive shelf at the implant
bone interface, the talar stem achieves stable fixation by engaging not only
the remaining body of the talus but also the inferior talar cortex, the superior calcaneal cortex, and the supportive cancellous bone in the calcaneus.
A stemmed tibial implant can provide stability by engaging the distal diaph-
yseal and metaphyseal bone. The stems and body sections are porous coated
to facilitate bony ingrowth. In many cases, the well-fixed tibial implant from
the original primary arthroplasty may be retained while the talar side is
revised, and the polyethylene liner exchanged.

The custom prosthesis is made from radiographs using standardized
radiographic template markers in the anteroposterior and lateral views,
which help determine the precise implant dimensions and stem angles.
The draft templates with these measurements are sent to the surgeon for
checking and approval before the fabrication process (Figs. 9–11). Generally, it takes about 6 weeks to have the custom component ready, which
must be taken into account in patient preparation and planning. The final
components are sterilized and individually packed. A stemless trial component with a guide channel for the stem preparation guidewire is made. Trial

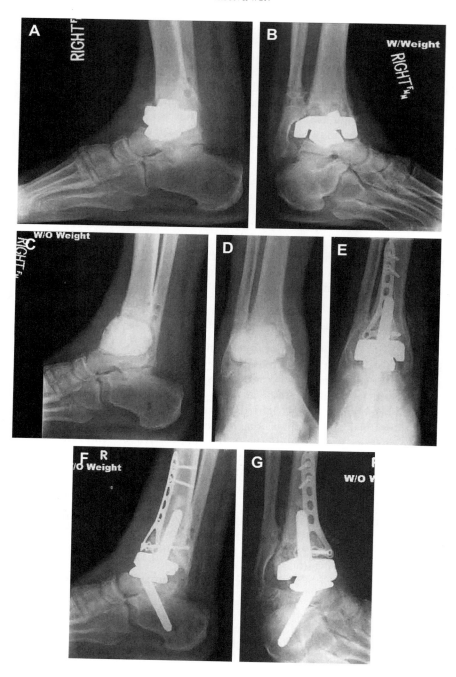

components of the same layout but with thinner stems (no porous coat) are also provided with the prosthesis to function as templates for insertion.

Surgical technique for revising agility total ankle replacement to custom prosthesis

Access to the joint should be by way of the previous longitudinal midline incision. If an alternative incision has been used that is not anatomically correct, care must be taken to decide on the correct course of the revision incision. If a talonavicular or a subtalar arthrodesis are to be performed simultaneously, then the incisions are planned accordingly to allow an adequate skin bridge on the lateral foot. Typically, the anterior central incision is used, and then as wide a skin bridge as possible is planned to include exposure of the subtalar joint. A short incision over the sinus tarsi is sufficient to expose the subtalar joint. Careful dissection is needed dorsally to minimize tissue trauma because this incision is prone to wound-healing complications. It can be difficult to separate the deep neurovascular bundle because of fibrosis and scarring, and the patient must be warned that dorsal foot numbness may occur if the deep or superficial peroneal nerve cannot be preserved.

Depending on the pathology, the implants may already be loose, or they may still be well fixed. The polyethylene insert is first removed from the tibial component to give more working space. Removal of the older versions of the polyethylene may be difficult because it is bottom loaded and will not slide out anteriorly until the edge rails are completely disengaged. If scarring is significant and the joint cannot be distracted, the polyethylene needs to be cut into segments with a reciprocating saw and removed piecemeal in large sections. Although destructive, it is the most efficient way of disrupting the edge-locking section of the older Agility poly tibial component. The polyethylene is generally easiest to remove once the talar component has been removed, which adds to the available room under the tibial component, and an osteotome can be inserted under the poly to lever it out. If it still seems too tight to remove the poly, then a laminar spreader can be inserted under the medial or lateral column of the tibial component, gaining more room to lever out the poly.

If the tibial component is stable and well positioned, it should not be revised. Because the newer Agility LP talar component has a different radius

Fig. 3. (A, B) This patient presented with infection 2.5 years after apparently successful ankle replacement. Note the bone lysis and component subsidence. (C, D) Treatment involved implant removal, antibiotic cement spacer, and systemic antibiotic therapy. After repeat debridement and treatment with another antibiotic spacer, the gram-negative infection was cleared. (E, F, G) The salvage procedure was performed with a long-stemmed tibial and talus, a cancellous bone graft, and a plate over the anterior tibia to keep the tibial cortical window in place during healing.

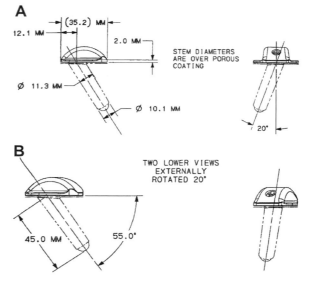

Fig. 4. (*A*) Custom talar prosthesis template with anteroposterior and lateral views relative to the dome of the implant. (*B*) Twenty degrees externally rotated views of the implant, corresponding with the appearance on standard anteroposterior and lateral radiographs of the ankle.

of curvature, a special mismatch polyethylene is required if an older version of the tibial component is retained, to articulate with the low profile talar component. One faces the same dilemma with reinsertion of the poly, which is bottom loading, so the poly has to be inserted before the talar component. One option here is to use a half column locking polyethylene liner for clearance, which can be slid under the tibial component without as much joint distraction. The side columns of the poly are not full length and are easier to insert. If the tibial component is unstable, loose, or malpositioned, it is

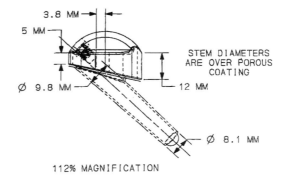

Fig. 5. Custom talar component with posteroinferior wedge augmentation to match the talar bone defect.

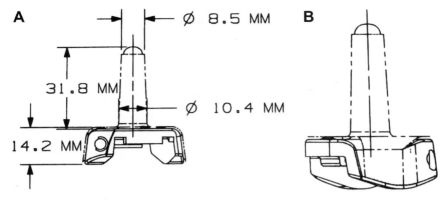

Fig. 6. (*A*) Anteroposterior and (*B*) lateral views of tibial stemmed custom component.

preferable to revise the whole tibial component to the low profile tibia, and the front-loading type of polyethylene liner can be used, which is much easier to insert. Removal of well-fixed components must be done meticulously, working at the interface with small, thin osteotomes to preserve as much bone as possible. Any overlying exostosis, debris, granulation, and scarred synovial tissue must be removed to aid visualization.

For the stemmed custom talar prosthesis, a formal subtalar arthrodesis is performed. The authors use a small 2-cm separate lateral incision over the inferior aspect of the sinus tarsi to prepare the joint surfaces. Debridement of the cartilage is performed with a rongeur and curved osteotomes, but the remaining talar and calcaneal subchondral bone must be preserved, and are perforated with a 2-mm drill. Once the arthroplasty components are inserted, screws are inserted to stabilize the subtalar joint. They are preferably inserted from the talar neck just distal to the talar component, aiming inferiorly into the calcaneus. The authors use two to three 3.5-mm screws to supplement the fixation by the component stem.

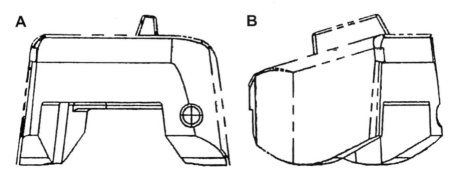

Fig. 7. (*A*) Anteroposterior and (*B*) lateral views of tibial component with angled base, functioning as wedge augmentation for bone defect.

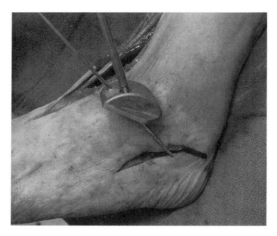

Fig. 8. A stemless trial talus with a tunnel in the body for a guidewire. The wire will direct the cannulated reamers to prepare the stem tunnel. Note the additional lateral incision for preparation of the subtalar joint.

The intraoperative sizing and tunnel preparation is done with a custom drill guide and trial component. The drill guide must be inserted into the talus and the calcaneus at the correct angle because this angle is preset in the long-stemmed talar component. The talar component should be parallel with the plane of the floor, or perpendicular to the long axis of the tibia. Because the trial talar component has a perforation to accommodate the

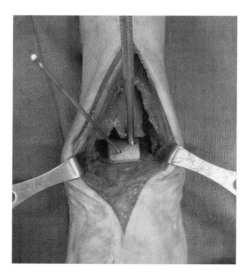

Fig. 9. Optimally positioned trial component with guidewire drilled into the calcaneus. The position is then confirmed on fluoroscopy.

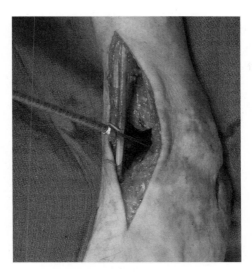

Fig. 10. The cannulated drill is used to prepare the stem tunnel. Note the screw at the talar neck supplementing the subtalar arthrodesis.

guide pin, the latter must be inserted at the correct angle. It is easiest to align the trial talus on the surface of the base of the remaining talus, but this alignment is not always possible because erosion of the remaining talar body may have occurred. If it is not possible to orient the base plate of the trial talar component flat with respect to the talus, then the guide must still be inserted to position the talar component parallel with the floor, and the anterior surface under the component filled with cancellous graft. The trial talus is positioned on the resected talar surface exactly as the final implant is to be oriented, including the built-in 20° of external rotation. It is best to confirm with fluoroscopy the correct position of the guide pin passing through the trial talar component.

The talar trial is removed while leaving the wire in situ. A graduated set of cannulated drills is used to enlarge the tunnel sequentially to the implant stem diameter. The custom trial component is then inserted to check if adequate diameter and length have been achieved. The stem of the actual component is slightly thicker because of the porous coat. The base of the talar component should be parallel with the floor. Despite careful preoperative planning and incorporating appropriately "built-in" wedge augmentations, intraoperative mismatch can still exist after debridement, which can create a problem if a large defect exists anteriorly between the base of the talar component and the calcaneus. Rather than leaving a defect, it should be filled with bone graft (Fig. 12).

After any necessary bone grafting, the authors have found it easiest to insert the stemmed talar component first, with the ankle in maximal plantar

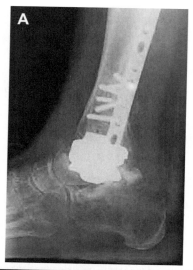

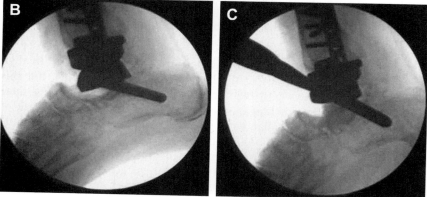

Fig. 11. (*A*) Preoperative lateral radiograph showing subsidence of talar component. The custom implant (from Fig. 6) was built with posteroinferior augmentation. Intraoperatively, the anterior talar bone defect was noted on the lateral fluoroscopy view after debridement. Note that the body of the talar component is parallel with the floor, leaving the anterior bone defect (*B*), which was filled with cancellous bone graft (*C*). (*D, E*) The final intraoperative fluoroscopic views. (*F, G*) Follow-up at 2 years showing stable components and 40° of ankle motion.

flexion, followed by the tibial component if it is revised. The polyethylene is installed last, unless it is a bottom-loading poly. Additional bone graft can still be packed in between the bone implant interface and squashed down. A mixture of cancellous bone graft with demineralized bone matrix is nicely malleable and sticky, so it does not become loose bodies in the joint. Final fluoroscopic screening is then performed to check that the implants have fully sealed. Also checked is range of motion. Further adjunctive procedures such as lengthening of the Achilles are sometimes needed.

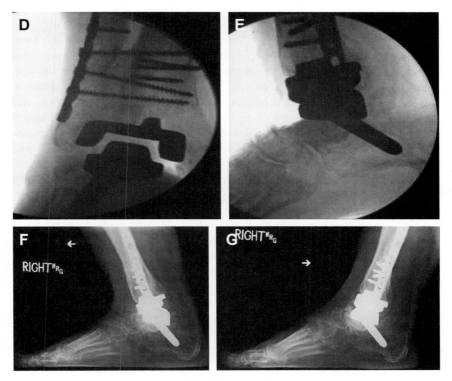

Fig. 11 (*continued*)

Postoperatively, rehabilitation is quicker for a custom revision than for primary arthroplasty. These long-stemmed implants are well fitted and, because the distal tibiofibular syndesmosis is fused, range of motion and bearing of weight can commence according to comfort. Patients are initially protected in a splint or cast for 2 weeks and, if the wound has healed, protected weight bearing is commenced with a removable boot.

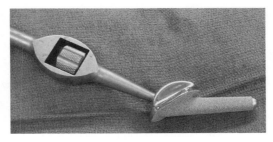

Fig. 12. The custom implant with inserter.

Tips and pitfalls

In planning for the revision, CT scans are helpful in assessing the local bone stock and the status of the adjacent joints. Visualizing the cystic and segmental defects can help plan bone grafting strategy and aid in implant choice and design. Standard primary components should be adequate if medial and lateral bone supports are present following bone resection and debridement. To ensure immediate stability and hence, facilitate adequate ingrowth, the contact surface area should have at least 50% healthy cancellous bone bed. If medial or lateral support is lacking, or if healthy bone bed contact is inadequate, then a stemmed custom implant should be used.

Despite careful planning, it is still possible to make errors in sizing and stem angulation, which makes actual implantation challenging. Also, no allowance exists for intraoperative changes of size, position, or alignment in cases where the bone resection level or bone quality may be different from the original plan. The authors would therefore advise having backup options available, which would consist of a full set of primary components and polyethylene liners of different thicknesses. A stemmed talar component is inserted most easily with the ankle maximally plantar flexed. One-piece stemmed tibial components are best inserted by way of an anterior distal tibial window (see Figs. 2 and 3). Custom components with long tibial stems can be made with a Morse taper junction with stem offset options to aid insertion in tight access situations and for fine tuning of alignment. It is to be hoped that more "off the shelf" modular components will be developed in the future to allow intraoperative adjustments.

Patients who have a coexisting pathology, such as subtalar joint arthritis or deformities in the hindfoot and midfoot, should have these pathologies addressed concurrently. As the prosthesis stem traverses the subtalar joint into the body of the calcaneus, it contributes to the fixation in adjunctive procedures like subtalar arthrodesis, calcaneal osteotomy, and triple arthrodesis performed in the same session. Additional hardware such as

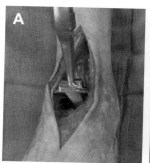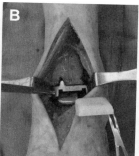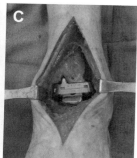

Fig. 13. (*A*) Implantation of talar component. (*B*) Implantation of tibial component. (*C*) The polyethylene liner is loaded anteriorly.

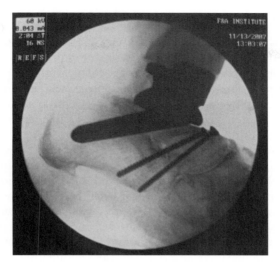

Fig. 14. Fluoroscopy is used liberally to check the position of implant, the screws, and the range of motion.

cannulated screws is invaluable and should be available. Plates and screws are likewise useful in securing any distal tibial cortical stem access windows. Availability of bone allograft is also handy in situations in which unexpected defects are encountered, for filling cysts, for use as structural graft under an implant, and less often, as a fall-back option for bone block arthrodesis (Figs. 13–15).

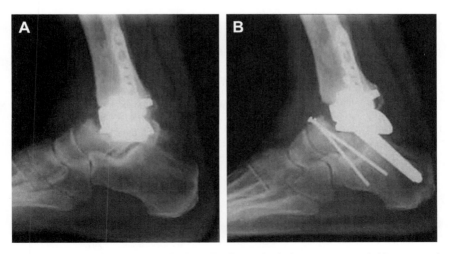

Fig. 15. (*A*) Pre- and (*B*) postoperative lateral radiograph of talar component subsidence treated with subtalar arthrodesis and a long-stemmed talar component. Note that the axis of the base of the talar component is parallel with the floor, although not perpendicular to the axis of the tibia.

Summary

With means for better mechanical stability and fixation, custom prostheses have improved our capabilities in salvaging failed total ankle replacements. Bone block arthrodesis is no longer the default end point. Mindful of the long-term problems of ankle, tibiotalocalcaneal, and more extensive arthrodesis, every effort must be made to restore physiologic function and maintain ankle motion. Even in the primary total ankle replacement setting, previous contraindications due to suboptimal bony support may be adequately bypassed, and more patients may benefit from having a custom prosthesis. To attain a successful outcome, careful workup is required, with consideration given to indications and contraindications. Accurate preoperative imaging and templating will ensure proper dimensions of the custom prosthesis. Intraoperative adjuncts like screws, plates, and bone grafts will help address unexpected bone defects, coexisting adjacent joint arthritis, and other hindfoot and midfoot deformities. Further research will help us to understand and work toward eliminating the causes and consequences of polyethylene particle osteolysis. The quest needs to continue to improve the longevity of total ankle replacements by reducing mechanical failures such as loosening and subsidence.

References

[1] Haddad SL, Coetzee JC, Estok R, et al. Intermediate and long-term outcomes of total ankle arthroplasty and ankle arthrodesis. A systematic review of the literature. J Bone Joint Surg Am 2007;89(9):1899–905.

[2] Knecht SI, Estin M, Callaghan JJ, et al. The agility total ankle arthroplasty. Seven to sixteen-year follow-up. J Bone Joint Surg Am 2004;86:1161–71.

[3] Conti SF, Wong YS. Complications of total ankle replacement. Foot Ankle Clin 2002;7(4): 791–807.

[4] Alvine FG. The agility ankle replacement: the good and the bad. Foot Ankle Clin 2002;7(4): 737–53, vi review.

[5] Doets HC, Brand R, Nelissen RG. Total ankle arthroplasty in inflammatory joint disease with use of two mobile-bearing designs. J Bone Joint Surg Am 2006;88:1272–84.

[6] San Giovanni TP, Keblish DJ, Thomas WH, et al. Eight-year results of a minimally constrained total ankle arthroplasty. Foot Ankle Int 2006;27(6):418–26.

[7] Kobayashi A, Minoda Y, Saltzman CL. Ankle arthroplasties generate wear particles similar to knee arthroplasties. Clin Orthop Relat Res 2004;424:69–72.

ELSEVIER
SAUNDERS

Foot Ankle Clin N Am
13 (2008) 539–547

FOOT AND
ANKLE CLINICS

Allograft Total Ankle Replacement—A Dead Ringer to the Natural Joint

Clifford L. Jeng, MD*, Mark S. Myerson, MD

Institute for Foot and Ankle Reconstruction, Mercy Medical Center, 301 St. Paul Place, Baltimore, MD 21202, USA

For decades, orthopedic surgeons have been looking for practical alternatives to ankle arthrodesis for the treatment of end-stage ankle arthritis. The desire to preserve ankle motion stems from the arthrodesis literature that shows long-term deficits in gait and the development of neighboring joint arthritis following fusion [1]. The most popular alternatives available today are total ankle replacement, supramalleolar osteotomy, and ankle distraction arthroplasty.

Fresh bipolar osteochondral allograft of the ankle joint has been sporadically reported in the literature as another alternative to ankle fusion. The theoretic advantage of this approach is that the ankle is biologically resurfaced with viable chondrocytes and a mature hyaline cartilage matrix. The chondrocytes are able to survive this transplantation process because cartilage is avascular and depends primarily on the surrounding synovial fluid for nutrition. These chondrocytes are also able to maintain the surrounding extracellular matrix. The underlying allograft bone that supports the cartilage subsequently heals to the host bone by creeping substitution [2].

This review of the current status of ankle transplantation first examines the basic science supporting the use of this technique. The five case series reported in the literature are discussed, followed by a description of the authors' preferred technique and short-term results.

Basic science

Fresh osteochondral transplants were performed in the knee for large focal defects and osteoarthritis long before they were attempted in the ankle

Dr. Jeng is a paid lecturer for DePuy Orthopaedics (Warsaw, Indiana) and has received research support from Smith & Nephew (Memphis, Tennessee).

* Corresponding author.

E-mail address: cjeng@mdmercy.com (C.L. Jeng).

joint. Because of this, most of the basic science literature that supports the use of fresh allografts comes from experience in the knee. Several concerns arise when discussing the transplantation of fresh cartilage tissue. One of the most important questions is whether chondrocytes can survive the transplantation process, particularly the cold-storage period. Several articles in the knee literature seem to indicate that they can survive these conditions well. One report harvested failed allografts at an average of 42 months and found 82% chondrocyte viability in the cartilage recovered [3]. Another study performed second-look biopsies of allograft cartilage and the surrounding host cartilage at 40 months after successful transplantation. The investigators found that the cell density and the viability of the transplanted chondrocytes were equivalent to that of the surrounding host cartilage [4]. Another important question is whether the original donor chondrocytes survive within the transplanted cartilage matrix long-term or whether they are eventually replaced with cells from the host. An interesting case report looked at a female donor knee allograft that was transplanted into a male recipient. Twenty-nine years after the initial transplant procedure, the allograft was removed before conversion to a total knee replacement. When the recovered allograft cartilage was examined, it was noted to have female XX chromosomes still present within the chondrocytes [5].

The mechanical properties of the cartilage extracellular matrix also appear to be well maintained during the transplantation process. Williams and colleagues [6] tested the biomechanical properties of osteochondral plugs from human femoral condyles stored for 28 days. There were no significant differences in glycosaminoglycan content, indentation stiffness, compressive modulus, permeability, or tensile modulus compared with initial values.

The underlying allograft bone that supports the cartilage heals to the host by creeping substitution. One study that analyzed failed osteochondral allografts after retrieval found that in 5 of 18 specimens, there was complete replacement of the allograft bone by host bone [2].

Much of the basic science research on osteochondral transplant has looked at optimal ways of storing and preparing allografts before implantation. Cold storage with fetal bovine serum added to the media increases chondrocyte viability and cell density compared with serum-free media. Proteoglycan synthesis in the allograft cartilage (measured by 35-sulfate radioactive tracer incorporation) is also increased with the inclusion of fetal bovine serum in the cold-storage media [7]. At the time of the transplant surgery, gradual rewarming of the allograft and treatment with a nitric oxide synthase inhibitor are beneficial in reversing the metabolic suppression that occurs during cold storage [8].

Several research studies have looked at the optimal window of time in which to transplant the fresh allografts before viability is significantly reduced. In human femoral condyle plugs stored in vitro for less than 14 days, there was no significant decline in chondrocyte viability or density.

After 28 days, however, there was a significant reduction in both of these measures [6]. In general, the loss of viable chondrocytes occurs in the critically important superficial zone of the cartilage [9]. An in vivo animal study looked at allograft osteochondral plugs transplanted into baboon knees. Allografts transplanted before 18 days of cold storage resulted in healthy cartilage at the time of sacrifice. Allografts transplanted after 21 days of cold storage resulted in cartilage that was pale, pitted, fragmented, and yellow. Histology of these specimens revealed absent chondrocytes [10].

The traditional teaching has been that cartilage is an immune-privileged tissue because of its avascularity. Chondrocytes themselves can be immunogenic, but they are protected from exposure to cytotoxic antibodies by the intact surrounding cartilage matrix. There is, however, an increasing body of evidence suggesting that this theory may be incorrect. Antibodies to cartilage-specific proteins were found in 57% of patients treated with fresh osteochondral allografts in the knee. The most common of the antibodies had molecular weights of 95 kd and 220 kd [11]. In the ankle joint, 91% of patients who underwent osteochondral allograft transplant had cytotoxic serum HLA antibodies at 6 months following implantation [12]. A radiologic study compared knee MRIs of osteochondral allograft patients who were serum antibody positive or antibody negative following surgery. The results showed that antibody-positive patients had greater bony edema in the transplanted allograft bone and the surrounding host bone. In addition, the graft–host interface was significantly wider in the antibody-positive individuals, indicative of less complete bony incorporation [13].

Review of literature

Gross and colleagues [14] were one of the earliest groups to report on the use of fresh osteochondral allograft tissue in the ankle. They performed unipolar transplants to the talus mostly for the treatment of osteochondritis dissecans lesions. Six of the nine allografts survived 11 years. The three failures were due to graft resorption and fragmentation. All three were revised to ankle arthrodesis.

Brage and colleagues [15] from University of California San Diego (UCSD) first presented the results of bipolar ankle transplantation in 2002. Sixteen patients underwent fresh cadaveric ankle transplantation and were followed for 62 months. There was an 87% allograft survival rate, with only three ankles requiring revision to an arthrodesis. The failures were due to graft fragmentation, graft subluxation, and nonunion. Kim and colleagues [16] later reported on the results of seven ankle transplants followed for 148 months at the same institution. They showed a 42% long-term failure rate. Allografts failed due to graft fragmentation, malunion, and nonunion. The patients' Short Form-12 general health survey scores at final follow-up were not significantly improved compared with preoperative values.

Due to the significant failure rates and the difficulty in precisely implanting the allografts using freehand saw cuts, the surgical technique was modified. The Agility total ankle replacement cutting jig (DePuy Orthopaedics, Inc., Warsaw, Indiana) was incorporated into the technique to help make more precise, matching cuts in the host and donor bones. Tontz and colleagues [17] from UCSD reviewed the results of 12 patients followed for 21 months using the newer technique. Nine patients had a bipolar tibiotalar allograft, 2 patients had a unipolar talar allograft, and 1 patient had a unipolar tibial allograft. Only one allograft (a partial unipolar allograft of the lateral talar dome) had to be revised due to graft collapse. The remaining 11 allografts were still in situ at the final follow-up.

Meehan and colleagues [12] followed 11 ankle transplants using the Agility cutting jig for an average of 33 months. Six of the 11 allografts survived, with a significant improvement in their American Orthopaedic Foot and Ankle Society (AOFAS) scores. Of the five failures, three underwent repeat allografting, one had a prosthetic total ankle replacement, and one was a radiographic failure but had not yet been revised. The patients in this series were tested for serum cytotoxic HLA antibodies. At 6 months postoperatively, 91% of the patients were positive for antibodies. The investigators speculated that the immune response of the host may play a more important role in fresh osteochondral allograft survival than previously believed.

The current literature on ankle transplantation is limited by the fact that all of the above studies are from a single institution (UCSD). Vora and Parks [18] were the first to report on a series of ankle transplants performed outside of UCSD. The study had 10 patients followed for a minimum of 1 year. Using a novel lateral transfibular approach and custom cutting jigs, they still noted a 50% failure rate of the allografts at final follow-up. Another limitation of the ankle transplant literature is that the follow-up has been relatively short in most of these case series.

Authors' surgical technique

The ankle joint is approached through an anterior midline incision. The interval between the extensor hallucis longus and tibialis anterior tendons is used. The neurovascular bundle is dissected out and retracted laterally. A synovectomy is performed to provide adequate visualization of the ankle joint. Anterior osteophytes are removed with an osteotome. The Agility total ankle replacement cutting jig is applied to the leg and the jig is affixed to the tibia after meticulously checking its position using intraoperative fluoroscopy. The distal tibial and medial malleolar cuts are made through the cutting jig with an oscillating saw, being careful to avoid fracturing the malleoli or injuring the neurovascular bundle. The flat talar dome cut is typically made through the inferior cutting jig. When the level of the cut appears too thick under fluoroscopic examination, however, the talar cut can be performed freehand.

The donor tibia is cut using the same-size Agility cutting jig. The allograft talus is cut freehand to match the thickness of the resected talus. The tibial and talar allografts are then inserted into the host ankle and placed through a range of motion to allow them to find their preferred position or "set point" within the ankle. The tibial allograft is fixed with two headless compression screws. The talar allograft is fixed with bioabsorbable pins. Ligamentous balancing is checked with varus and valgus stressing of the ankle under fluoroscopy. If any instability exists, it is addressed with collateral ligament releases or with ligament reconstruction. The ankle joint capsule is meticulously closed, followed by skin closure.

Following surgery, the ankle is protected in a bulky Jones compressive bandage with plaster splints for 2 weeks until the incision is healed. At that point, the ankle is placed in a removable cam boot, and patients are encouraged to perform active range-of-motion exercises out of the boot at home, independently. Formal therapy is usually started at 6 weeks postoperatively, and patients are kept non–weight bearing for 12 weeks. The cam boot is typically discontinued at 12 weeks following surgery, and patients are then transferred to an air stirrup ankle brace. In cases in which there is a delayed union of the allograft to the host bone, patients are immobilized for longer periods. Physical therapy is continued for an additional 1 to 3 months. Low-impact exercises such as swimming and using the treadmill and stationary bike and are encouraged at this point; however, high-impact activities are prohibited for the first year following surgery.

Results

Twenty-nine patients underwent bipolar osteochondral allograft of the ankle joint at the authors' institution between 2003 and 2005. The mean age of this patient group was 41 years (range, 18–57 years). The mean duration of follow-up was 2 years (range, 11–35 months). There were 15 men and 14 women in this series.

Data collected pertaining to the donor included the donor's age and time from asystole to implantation of the graft. Characteristics of the transplant recipient that were analyzed included the patient's age, body mass index, and the preoperative radiographic ankle alignment. Factors related to the surgical procedure itself that were assessed included the thickness of the tibial and talar allografts and the postoperative radiographic ankle alignment obtained following surgery.

At the final follow-up, all 29 patients were available for evaluation. With removal of the allograft as the end point, there were 15 successful transplants and 14 failures, resulting in a survival rate of 51.7% at 24 months. Six transplants in this series, however, had radiographic evidence of allograft failure but had not yet been revised. Evidence of radiographic failure included graft fracture, graft collapse, or loss of joint space. If these 6 patients who had radiographic failures were added to the 14 allografts that were revised, then there was a total of 9 successes and 20 failures, giving an overall survival rate of 31% at 2 years.

The mode of allograft failure was as follows. There were six tibial allograft fractures and two talar allograft fractures. Five patients developed isolated collapse of the tibial side of the allograft. Six patients developed loss of joint space and end-stage arthritis. One patient developed a deep infection requiring removal of the ankle transplant. There were no nonunions at the host–graft interface on the tibial side or the talar side of the transplant.

Of the 14 failed allografts that required revision, 5 underwent repeat osteochondral ankle transplantation. Three patients were converted to an Agility total ankle replacement. Five patients were revised to an ankle arthrodesis with an interposition femoral head allograft. The patient who had the deep infection eventually obtained a successful fusion with an external fixator following removal of the allograft and multiple debridements.

The five patients who underwent repeat ankle transplant following an initial failed allograft were reviewed. Two are doing well with satisfactory radiographs and no clinical complaints. One has developed narrowing of the joint space with some painful symptoms, but is still better off than after the first transplant. Of the remaining two patients, one has been converted to a prosthetic total ankle replacement and the other has been converted to a bone block ankle fusion.

The nine successful ankle allografts were evaluated for clinical range of motion and AOFAS ankle-hindfoot scores at final follow-up. The average range of motion preoperatively was 25°(3° dorsiflexion, 22° plantarflexion). The average postoperative range of motion was 21° (3° dorsiflexion, 18° plantarflexion). There was no significant difference between preoperative and postoperative motion.

The average AOFAS ankle-hindfoot score was 84 (range, 71–96) at final follow-up. The average for the pain component of the AOFAS score was 31 out of a possible 40. The average for the function component of the AOFAS score was 44 out of a possible 50. No preoperative scores were available for comparison. When the nine successful allograft patients were asked whether they would undergo the procedure again, 67% responded yes, 11% responded no, and 22% were unsure.

The average age of the patients in the success group was 45.7 years versus 38.4 years in the failure group. The average body mass index of the patients in the success group was 24.3 versus 28.4 in the failure group. These differences were statistically significant ($P = .04$ and .02, respectively).

Radiographs of the patients in this series were analyzed preoperatively and postoperatively at each follow-up visit. There was significantly less preoperative ankle deformity in the coronal plane in the success group compared with the failure group (2.4° versus 5.8°); however, there was no difference between the two groups with respect to the postoperative ankle alignment achieved after surgery or the thickness of the tibial or talar allografts implanted.

Other factors not found to be significantly different between the success and failure groups were the donor's age and the time from death of the donor to implantation.

Summary

The authors' series of ankle transplants is the largest reported in the literature to date. Compared with the articles from the UCSD group, however, the allograft survival rate is conspicuously lower in this series. Probably the most significant difference between the authors' experience and UCSD's is the time from donor asystole to implantation of the allograft. In the four reports from UCSD, the average time from death of the donor to implantation was 5 to 7 days compared with 23 days in the current series [12,15–17]. This time difference is largely due to a recent change in the tissue bank industry standards that now requires a minimum of 14 days of microbiologic testing before the harvested allografts are declared sterile and released for implantation. As demonstrated in multiple in vitro research studies, there are significant adverse effects of prolonged cold storage on chondrocyte viability in these allografts.

There are some subtle differences in surgical technique between the patients in this series and the protocol described in the UCSD articles. Brage and colleagues [15] used an external fixator to distract the tibiotalar joint and to realign any ankle deformity before making saw cuts. This technique may theoretically provide a more well balanced ankle joint following implantation. The UCSD group also described using an Agility cutting jig for the donor tibia that is one size larger than the jig used to resect the host tibia. This difference in jig size likely results in a thicker tibial graft that may better resist fracture later. Finally, they routinely lavaged the bone marrow elements from the allograft before implantation, which may potentially decrease the possibility of transplanting immunogenic factors leading to graft failure.

Meehan and colleagues [12] stated that the main risk factors for ankle transplant failure are size mismatch between the donor and the recipient and cutting the tibial or talar allograft excessively thin. In the current series, the authors were also concerned about their patients in whom the tibial or talar grafts were implanted too thin. There were two tibial allografts and one talar allograft measuring less than 0.65 cm in thickness in the authors' study. Although each of these allografts subsequently fractured in the early postoperative period, the authors were unable to show graft thickness as an independent predictor of failure, most likely because of the small number of patients in the study.

The factors found to be significantly different between the success group and the failure group were the recipient's body mass index, the recipient's age, and the magnitude of preoperative ankle malalignment. Ankle transplants performed in hosts who had a low body mass index and less preoperative deformity and who were older were more likely to survive. It may be difficult to interpret the actual clinical importance of these criteria, however, due to the subtle differences in the numbers and the overall high failure rate in this series.

The factors not found to be statistically different between the success group and the failure group were the donor's age, the time from death of the donor to implantation, the thickness of the tibial and talar allografts, and the postoperative radiographic ankle alignment.

The continued use of ankle transplantation as an alternative to ankle arthrodesis for the treatment of end-stage ankle arthritis should be viewed with some skepticism. In this series of 29 patients, there was a prohibitively high failure rate, and salvage of failed allografts has proved to be extremely challenging. The authors currently consider this procedure at their institution only in patients who are too young for prosthetic ankle replacement; in those who have excellent ankle range of motion, low body mass index, and normal radiographic alignment; and in those who refuse an ankle arthrodesis.

References

[1] Coester LM, Saltzman CL, Leupold J, et al. Long-term results following ankle arthrodesis for post-traumatic arthritis. J Bone Joint Surg Am 2001;83:219–28.
[2] Oakeshott RD, Farine I, Pritzker KP, et al. A clinical and histologic analysis of failed fresh osteochondral allografts. Clin Orthop Relat Res 1988;233:283–94.
[3] Williams SK, Amiel D, Ball ST, et al. Analysis of cartilage tissue on a cellular level in fresh osteochondral allograft retrievals. Am J Sports Med 2007;35:2022–32.
[4] Davidson PA, Rivenburgh DW, Dawson PE, et al. Clinical, histologic, radiographic outcomes of distal femoral resurfacing with hypothermically stored osteoarticular allografts. Am J Sports Med 2007;35:1082–90.
[5] Jamali Amir A, Hatcher Sandra L, You Zongbing. Donor cell survival in a fresh osteochondral allograft at twenty-nine years. A case report. J Bone Joint Surg Am 2007;89:166–9.
[6] Williams SK, Amiel D, Ball ST, et al. Prolonged storage effects on the articular cartilage of fresh human osteochondral allografts. J Bone Joint Surg Am 2003;85:2111–20.
[7] Pennock AT, Wagner F, Robertson CM, et al. Prolonged storage of osteochondral allografts: does the addition of fetal bovine serum improve chondrocyte viability? J Knee Surg 2006;19:265–72.
[8] Pylawka TK, Virdi AS, Cole BJ, et al. Reversal of suppressed metabolism in prolonged cold preserved cartilage. J Orthop Res 2008;26:247–54.
[9] Allen RT, Robertson CM, Pennock AT, et al. Analysis of stored osteochondral allografts at the time of surgical implantation. Am J Sports Med 2005;33:1479–84.
[10] Malinin T, Temple HT, Buck BE. Transplantation of osteochondral allografts after cold storage. J Bone Joint Surg Am 2006;88:762–70.
[11] Phipatanakul WP, VandeVord PJ, Teitge RA, et al. Immune response in patients receiving fresh osteochondral allografts. Am J Orthop 2004;33:345–8.
[12] Meehan R, McFarlin S, Bugbee W, et al. Fresh ankle osteochondral allograft transplantation for tibiotalar joint arthritis. Foot Ankle Int 2005;26:795–802.
[13] Sirlin CB, Brossmann J, Boutin RD, et al. Shell osteochondral allografts of the knee: comparison of MR imaging findings and immunologic responses. Radiology 2001;219: 35–43.

[14] Gross AE, Agnidis Z, Hutchison CR. Osteochondral defects of the talus treated with fresh osteochondral allograft transplantation. Foot Ankle Int 2001;22:385–91.

[15] Brage ME, Bugbee W, Tontz W. Intraoperative and postoperative complications of fresh tibiotalar allografting. Presented at the AOFAS Winter Meeting. Dallas, TX, February 16, 2002.

[16] Kim CW, Jamali A, Tontz W, et al. Treatment of post-traumatic ankle arthrosis with bipolar tibiotalar osteochondral shell allografts. Foot Ankle Int 2002;23:1091–102.

[17] Tontz W, Bugbee W, Brage M. Use of allografts in the management of ankle arthritis. Foot Ankle Clin 2003;8:361–73.

[18] Vora A, Parks B. Early failure of bipolar osteochondral tibiotalar allograft replacements. Presented at the AOFAS Winter Meeting. Washington, DC, February 26, 2005.

ELSEVIER
SAUNDERS

Foot Ankle Clin N Am
13 (2008) 549–570

FOOT AND
ANKLE CLINICS

Index

Note: Page numbers of article titles are in **boldface** type.

1083-7515/08/$ - see front matter © 2008 Elsevier Inc. All rights reserved.
doi:10.1016/S1083-7515(08)00060-0